ADOLESCENT PREGNANCY PREVENTION

A GUIDEBOOK FOR COMMUNITIES

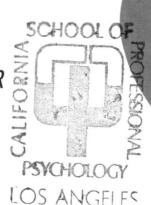

by

CLAIRE D. BRINDIS

with

KAREN PITTMAN

PATRICIA REYES

SHARON ADAMS-TAYLOR

HEALTH PROMOTION RESOURCE CENTER
Stanford Center for Research in Disease Prevention
In Cooperation with The Henry J. Kaiser Family Foundation

Health Promotion Resource Center
Stanford Center for Research in Disease Prevention,
1000 Welch Road, Palo Alto, CA 94304-1885

Adolescent Pregnancy Prevention: A Guidebook for Communities
was developed under a grant from the Henry J. Kaiser Family Foundation.

The mention of trade names, commercial products or organizations does not imply
endorsement by Stanford University nor by the funders of this project.

ISBN 1-879552-00-0

Table of Contents

Acknowledgements   *xv*

Introduction   *xix*

Section I   **A Profile of Teenage Pregnancy**
                     Prevention Programs   1

Chapter 1   **A Conceptual Framework for Understanding**
                     Adolescent Pregnancy   3

• Framing the Problem and the Solution

What Can We Learn from Research?   4

• The Reproductive Continuum

• Breaking Down Teen Births into Categories

• Trends in Teenage Reproductive Behavior

• Targeting the Boys

Predictors of Early Sexual Activity, Contraceptive Use,
Pregnancy, and Parenthood   8

• Related Problem Behaviors

Providing Teens with the Capacity to Prevent Pregnancy   10

• Sexuality and Family Life Education

• Contraceptive Services

• Sexually Transmitted Disease Services

• Abortion Services

Creating the Opportunity Structure to Prevent Pregnancy   **12**

• Enhanced Education

• Employment Potential

• Social Support

• Key Factors in Successful Programs

Summary   **14**

Appendix 1-1   **Adolescent Pregnancy and Parenting Fact Sheet**   **15**

References   **20**

Chapter 2   **Preventing Teenage Pregnancy:**
Creating the Capacity and the Opportunity Structure   **23**

Building the Capacity to Prevent Teenage Pregnancy   **25**

• Information and Counseling

Programs and Curricula   **27**

• Family Life/Sex Education Curricula

• Abstinence Curricula

• Life Planning and Life Skills

• Improving Parent/Child Communication

• Individual and Small-group Counseling

• System-wide Programs

• Contraceptive Counseling and Services

• Linking Capacity-building Information With Contraceptive Services

• Comprehensive Adolescent Health Clinics

Enhancing Life Options: Creating the Opportunity
Structure to Prevent Teenage Pregnancy   **38**

• Linking Family Life Education to Life Options Programs

• Comprehensive Programs to Improve Life Options

Implications for Program Development
and Community-wide Planning   **41**

Summary   **42**

Appendix 2-1   **Model Adolescent Pregnancy Prevention Programs**   **43**

Chapter 3   **Community-wide Interventions and Resources for Support   47**

Resources   **48**

- Funding for Family Life and Sex Education
- Funding for Pregnancy Prevention Programs and Contraception
- Funding for Life Options
- Funding for Health Services
- Funding for Substance Abuse
- Efforts at the State Level

Community-wide Pregnancy Prevention Initiatives   **53**

- Key Ingredients
- Mayor's Office of Adolescent Pregnancy
  and Parenting Services, New York City
- Planned Parenthood of East Central Georgia Program,
  Jasper County, South Carolina
- IMPACT 88: County-wide Plan for Reducing
  Teen Pregnancy, Dallas, Texas
- Life Options Coalition, Milwaukee, Wisconsin
- Committee on Adolescent Pregnancy and
  Parenting (CAPP), Minneapolis Public Schools
- The New Futures Initiative: The Annie E. Casey Foundation
- The Montana Coalition of Healthy Mothers, Healthy Babies:
  Promoting Action forTeen Health (PATH) Project

Summary   **76**

Section II   **How to Develop a Community-wide
                 Adolescent Pregnancy Prevention Initiative   77**

Chapter 4   **Getting Started: The Coalition and the Lead Agency   79**

**Putting Together a Broad-based Coalition
for Pregnancy Prevention**   **80**

Structure of a Community-wide Coalition   **80**

Demonstrating Community-wide Support   **82**

The Steering Committee or Board of Directors   85

Designating a Lead Agency   87

The Role of a Lead Agency   88

The Role of the Coordinator   89

Making Coalition Meetings Work   89

Facing Controversy   89

After You Are Organized   90

• Establishing a Set of Community Standards – How to Create Consensus

• Sample Standards for Program Development: Potential Roles
  of Community Agencies in Adolescent Pregnancy Prevention

• Community and Agency Standards

Summary   96

Appendix 4-1   The Initial Planning Meeting   97

Appendix 4-2   A Coalition-building Checklist   103

Appendix 4-3   Decision-making Approaches for Your Board and Coalition   107

Chapter 5   Needs Assessment and Data Collection   113

What is a Needs Assessment?   114

Why do a Community-wide Needs Assessment?   114

Interorganizational Relationships   115

Consider Your Goals   116

What is the Target Community?   116

Estimating Unmet Need   117

Getting Started   118

The Scope of Your Assessment   118

• A Road Map

• Examples of Needs Assessment Questions

• Demographic Profile

• Community Resources

• Adolescents at Risk of Pregnancy and Other Risk Behaviors

• General Information Questions to Ask All Providers

Sources of Needs Assessment Data   124

• Public Documents and Statistics

• Other Sources of Community Information

Developing Your Information Matrix   129

• Preparing the Questions

Developing a Workplan   130

• Training Interviewers

• Deciding Whom to Interview

• Protection of Human Rights

• Building Trust

The Needs Assessment Report   132

• Using Needs Assessment Data to Increase Interagency Cooperation

• Preparing and Disseminating Your Report

Next Steps   134

Summary   135

Appendix 5-1   **A Guide for Calculating a Community's Birthrate**   137

Appendix 5-2   **Needs Assessment Data Collection Guide**   139

Chapter 6   **Utilizing Needs Assessment Data
                to Create an Implementation Plan**   153

                Selecting Planning Areas   154

                Defining the Target Population   155

Assessing the Expansion Potential of Existing Programs   **160**

Setting Priorities for Facility Expansion   **161**
- Integration of New Efforts Within the Established Network
- Location in Relation to Concentration(s) of Youths in Need
- Access to Care

Sample Plans   **165**

Structure for Coordinating Functions   **167**
- Functions That Can Be Performed by a Community-wide Coordinating Agency or Group
- Organizational Structures

The Implementation Plan   **172**
- Gaining Community Support
- Formulating Goals and Objectives
  1. Coordination of Services Among Community Programs
  2. Program Planning and Development
  3. Community Awareness and Commitment to Community-based Adolescent Pregnancy Prevention Efforts
  4. Coordination of Funding

Summary   **176**

Appendix 6-1   **Data on Sexual Activity**   **177**

Appendix 6-2   **Primary Goals and Strategies**   **179**

Appendix 6-3   **Calculating Staff Time Requirements**   **181**

Chapter 7   **Implementing Community Strategies**   **183**

The Implementation Committee   **183**
- Establishing a Time Line

Strengthening Collaboration   **184**

Implementing Interagency Coordination   **185**

Exploring Outside Resources   **186**

Initiating Interagency Activities   **187**

- Fostering Cooperation
- Formal Agreements
- Meeting Client Needs through Effective Referrals
- Ways to Decrease Service Fragmentation
- Ways to Increase Accessibility of Client Services
- Development of a Coalition Information Clearinghouse
- Joint Program Design
- Joint Budgeting
- Personnel

The Media Link   **194**

- Dissemination of the Implementation Plan

Planning for Long-term Funding   **197**

Potential Sources of Funding   **199**

- Private Sources
- Public Sources
- Locating Public Funding Sources
- In-kind Services

Developing A Budget   **202**

Proposal Writing   **203**

- Key Proposal Ingredients

Be Prepared to Revise the Implementation Plan   **205**

Summary   **205**

Appendix 7-1   **Force Field Analysis**   **207**

Appendix 7-2   **What You Can Gain or Provide
Through Interagency Coordination**   **211**

Chapter 8   **Evaluating the Community-wide Plan**   **213**

Types of Evaluation   **214**

What Should You Evaluate? 217

- Process Objectives
- Outcome Objectives
- Impact Objectives

Who Should Evaluate? 219

Planning an Evaluation 220

Evaluation Manual 221

Steps in the Evaluation Process 222

Step 1: Review Needs Assessment 222

Step 2: State Measurable Objectives 223

- Formula for Stating Objectives

Step 3: Identify Resources and Constraints 224

Step 4: Specify What Information is to be Collected 227

- Information To Be Collected for the Community-wide Evaluation

Step 5: Choose the Evaluation Design 231

- Post-assessment Only
- One-group Pre- and Post-assessment
- Pre-test/Post-test Comparison Group
- Time Series Design
- Establishing a Control or Comparison Group
- Random Assignment

Step 6: Choose the Data Collection Method 236

- Questionnaires and Surveys
- Using Existing Questionnaires
- Principles for Writing Good Questionnaires
- Interviews
- Existing Program Records
- Public Records
- Observations

Step 7: Test and Refine Procedures and Tools 248

Step 8: Collect Data 248

- Confidentiality of Data

Step 9: Analyze Data   249
- Descriptive Analysis
- Summarizing Open-ended Questions
- Preparing the Results for Presentation

Step 10: Report Findings   255
- Components of the Report

Step 11: Act on Findings   256
- Program Feedback and Improvement
- Assessing Impact of Program
- Program Planning
- Complying with Program Requirements

Summary   257

Appendix 8-1   Using A Random Numbers Table   259

General Resource Directory   261

Organizations   261

Topical Bibliography   268
- Abortion
- Adolescent Males and Teen Pregnancy
- Adolescent Pregnancy
- Adolescent Pregnancy Prevention
- AIDS and Sexually Transmitted Diseases
- Controversial Issues
- Development and Evaluation of Programs
- Family Life Education
- Family Planning
- Funding
- School-based Health Clinics

Additional Resources   273

Bibliography   275

Table of Charts and Worksheets

Chart 1-1	A Snapshot Profile of 15-19-Year-Old Teenage Women in 1985	5
Chart 1-2	Births to women younger than 20	7
Chart 3-1	Community-wide Pregnancy Prevention Initiative	48
Chart 4-1	Development of an Organizational Structure	81
Chart 4-2	Examples of Agencies and Individuals to Include in a Broad-based Coalition on Adolescent Pregnancy Prevention	83
Chart 4-3	The Program-planning Process	91
Chart 5-1	Developing a Demographic Profile of Adolescent Pregnancy in the Community	121
Chart 6-1	Planning Overview	159
Chart 6-2	Expansion Potential of Existing Facilities	159
Chart 6-3	Priority Ratings for Anytown's Program Sites	163
Chart 6-4	Coordinating Organization Structure: Separate Coalition Model, Divided Functions by Organization	171
Chart 6-5	Coordinating Organization Structure: Separate Coalition Model	171
Chart 6-6	Components of Community-wide Teen Pregnancy Prevention Effort	175
Worksheet 4-1	Planning for the First Meeting	101
Worksheet 4-2	A Coalition-building Checklist	103
Worksheet 5-1	Needs Assessment Questions	149
Worksheet 5-2	Sources of Data for the Needs Assessment	150
Worksheet 5-3	Needs Assessment Matrix	151
Worksheet 6-1	Anytown Family Planning Service Profile to Document Adolescents in Need of Family Planning Services	157
Worksheet 7-1	What Do You Know About Other Agencies?	189

Worksheet 7-2   What You Can Gain or Provide Through Interagency Coordination   211

Worksheet 8-1   Identifying Resources and Constraints   226

Worksheet 8-2   Sample Participant Summary Form   228

Worksheet 8-3   Identifying Methods of Data Collection   237

Worksheet 8-4   Case Management Project: Chart Review   245

Acknowledgements

*T*his guidebook builds upon the collective experience of many health and social service professionals, program managers, and community leaders committed to improving the status of young people in our society. It is with the sincerest gratitude that I extend my appreciation to my co-authors: Karen Pittman, who at the time this guidebook was written was Director of the Adolescent Pregnancy Prevention/Education Division at the Children's Defense Fund, Washington, D.C.; Patricia Reyes, Research Associate at the Center for Reproductive Health Policy Research, Institute for Health Policy Studies, University of California, San Francisco; and Sharon Adams-Taylor, who at the time this guidebook was written was Senior Program Associate of the Adolescent Pregnancy Prevention/Education Division, Children's Defense Fund, Washington, D.C. Ms. Pittman is currently at the Academy for Educational Development in Washington, D.C. and Ms. Adams-Taylor is at the American Association of School Administrators in Arlington, Virginia.

Ms. Pittman and Ms. Adams-Taylor were the principal authors of the first two chapters of the book, which discuss the antecedents and outcomes of adolescent pregnancy, community-wide intervention strategies, and the background for our present overall conceptualization of the problem. In addition to this major contribution, they also provided invaluable feedback to me on the other chapters in the book throughout the many stages of its writing, from original drafts to the completed manuscript. It is no exaggeration to say that their breadth of knowledge and their commitment to the improvement of overall child and adolescent health and the development of community-wide adolescent pregnancy prevention efforts have been a wellspring of inspiration for me.

Patricia Reyes, my valued colleague at the Center for Reproductive Health Policy Research, conducted extensive interviews with community representatives highlighted in the case studies in Chapter 3 and was responsible for the initial drafting of several chapters. In addition to conducting much of the background research that I relied upon throughout the volume, she provided ongoing assistance and support during its development that helped move the book closer to its goal of giving practical community guidance.

I am grateful as well to many other individuals whose experience and expertise have been incorporated into this volume. In particular, I am deeply indebted to Joy Dryfoos, whose writings and thoughtful comments greatly contributed to both the background and the planning chapters in this volume. Ms. Dryfoos' longtime commitment to and broad study of family planning have been a shaping force at several important junctures in the emergence of this young field. Her pioneering work was responsible for developing the first formulas and planning guides used by communities to determine the numbers of women in need of family planning services. Many of the tenets of the planning guidelines she has developed are as applicable today as they were when first conceptualized nearly twenty years ago and continue to be applicable to diverse social issues, as is evident in this volume. Her leadership has been in great part responsible for crystallizing our current approach to the prevention of early childbearing: the need for services to expand life options for young people and enhance their capacity to deal with their sexuality in a responsible manner, including increased access to contraceptive care. We believe that these key factors serve to increase young people's motivation to avoid premature pregnancy. This synthesis of ideas and concepts represents the underlying philosophy of this book.

I am also grateful to Philip R. Lee, M.D., Professor of Social Medicine and Director of the Institute for Health Policy Studies, University of California, San Francisco, whose mentoring, personal support, and strong commitment to the field of reproductive health policy helped create the professional and collegial environment in which this volume was written. Several members of the Institute's administrative staff also provided invaluable assistance, particularly Nancy Ramsay, who worked diligently to edit the manuscript and provide the clarity essential to ensure that this guidebook will fulfill its purpose. Her guidance and expertise have greatly contributed to this volume. The joint and dedicated efforts of Steve Guinn, Eunice Chee, and Steve Snider were responsible for the arduous task of manuscript preparation. I would also like to acknowledge the contribution made by Madeline Stanionis, one of the Center's fine research assistants, who spent many hours on the telephone compiling and verifying information for the book's resource directory.

Special thanks must also go to Todd Rogers, Ph.D., David Altman, Ph.D., and Nancy Houston Miller, R.N., of the Stanford Health Promotion Resource Center, who first helped to conceptualize the book and who recognized the necessity of developing a guidebook that would be applicable to communities across the country. I am particularly grateful to Dr. Altman for his vital ongoing support throughout the many months between the project's initial conceptualization and its final realization. The excellent editorial and production assistance of Prudence Breitrose, M.A., and David Collins of the Stanford Health Promotion Resource Center also helped bring this project to fruition. In addition, I am thankful to the Henry J. Kaiser Family Foundation for its financial support and sponsorship of this effort, as well as for its dedication to improving the quality of life in communities across the country.

My sincere appreciation also goes to Sharon Lovick, Amy Loomis, and Michelle Cahill for their comments during the final stages of the book's preparation. Their review of this work has helped to ensure that its contents will provide some guidance to communities and concerned individuals who are striving to mitigate the adverse effects of inadequate programs for children and adolescents. And finally, a heartfelt word of appreciation to my husband Ralph and our sons Seth and Daniel, whose love and support have encouraged and sustained me during this project, and indeed, in all my work.

Claire Brindis, Dr.P.H.
Center for Reproductive Health Policy Research
Institute for Health Policy Studies
Department of Pediatrics, Division of Adolescent Medicine
University of California, San Francisco

Introduction

The United States has the highest teenage pregnancy rate of any developed nation, with approximately one million teenage pregnancies annually. Nearly half of these pregnancies result in the birth of a child, and almost all these young mothers choose to keep the child in their home. Adolescent childbearing has become a pressing social issue because of its broad social and economic consequences for the mothers, their families, the babies, and for society. The negative effects of early childbearing affect the health, education, and employment opportunities of the mothers; poverty is a frequent outcome. The long-term implications for the offspring include poor opportunities in society, risks of poor health, and adverse developmental outcomes.

Although adolescents today are maturing earlier, the time between development of their ability to reproduce and the time of full adulthood, when they are equipped with the means to support and maintain a family, is considerable. Our complex society requires long years of training and preparation for individuals to obtain the requisite skills to take on the psychological, financial, and social responsibilities of childbearing. Yet, alarmingly, births to younger adolescents have escalated in recent years, and the proportion of unmarried adolescent mothers is also growing. As these teenage mothers drop out of school with relatively few skills, they place great financial burdens on society for many years to come.

Although programs do exist to assist adolescents in postponing pregnancy, they reach only a limited group and often provide inadequate support. The diversity among adolescents and in their needs for assistance requires that multiple strategies be developed offering both comprehensive and diversified resources targeted at appropriate intervention points along the continuum of teenage life.

Ample evidence exists from the experiences of other developed nations to show that early sexual activity need not necessarily result in high pregnancy and birth rates. Despite rates of sexual activity that are similar to those among U.S. teenagers, most Western nations have considerably lower pregnancy and abortion rates. In contrast to the United States, other industrialized nations such as Canada, Sweden, France, the Netherlands, and the United Kingdom, have a wider acceptance of sexual activity among young people by parents and other adults, and in turn a more responsible attitude toward sexuality and its consequences by teenagers. This results in much more effective use of contraception by teens who are sexually active.

Rates of adolescent pregnancy are one important indicator of a nation's well-being, and our high rate of teenage pregnancy and childbearing is a symptom of major social and economic ills. No cure can be expected unless underlying causes such as poverty, lack of education, isolation, low self-esteem, and lack of hope are addressed through well-coordinated efforts involving public and private services at many levels.

Causes of Teen Pregnancy

More than one in ten U.S. teenage girls has become pregnant every year for the past decade. There is general agreement that society should implement strategies to address this issue, but little agreement exists about the actual causes of teen pregnancy. Many divergent factors are postulated:

- **"Too early intercourse."** (Young people should not engage in premarital sexual relations. Early sexual activity reflects permissiveness and a lack of morality in the society at large and a decline of the American family as the guiding force in moral development.)

- **"Lack of knowledge."** (Young people do not know enough about their bodies, reproductive processes, nor how to prevent pregnancy. They are not aware of the risk of pregnancy nor of the consequences of early childbearing.)

- **"Lack of skills in decision-making and communication."** (Teenagers do not know how to resist the pressures that arise in peer situations; they fear the rejection that might result from not going along with the crowd.)

- **"Lack of access to contraception."** (Even where family planning clinics exist, teenagers do not feel comfortable using them. Some are afraid because of real or imagined parental notification rules; others cannot afford the fees.)

- **"Lack of access to abortion services."** (Because of cost, parental consent policies, lack of pregnancy counseling and other barriers, access to abortion services can be limited.)

- **"Lack of attention to males."** (While boys also suffer from lack of access to contraception counseling and services, knowledge, and skills, their needs are rarely addressed.)

- **"Fewer marriages and fewer adoptions."** (There have always been teenage mothers; the problem is that today, young girls are not marrying when faced with an unintended pregnancy, nor are they giving their children up for adoption as frequently as in the past.)

- **"Lack of opportunity."** (With few perceived options in society, disadvantaged youngsters are not motivated to delay parenthood. While most teen pregnancies are unintentional, teens from low socioeconomic backgrounds believe that childbearing will not negatively affect their future status, and so they drift into parenthood.)

- **"Welfare."** (The system rewards young women for becoming mothers, particularly those who are eager to leave home and set up their own households.)

- **"The media."** (By depicting sexually explicit material and not providing young people with responsible role models, print and electronic media convey a confusing message about appropriate behavior for young people. There is also an absence of birth control in the popular media, particularly television and movies.)

In reality, the problem results from a combination of all these themes. While achieving complete consensus on the solutions to such an array of issues may be impossible, each problem listed above must be addressed and decisions made about its resolution.

This guidebook is aimed at helping groups assess which issues or factors need to be addressed in their community, what resources are needed and available, and what interventions will be most successful in achieving local objectives. It is the authors' hope that a careful reading of this manual will result in a decision to view teen pregnancy prevention rationally and comprehensively and ultimately lead to plans based on factual information rather than on ideologies and illusion.

Ideas presented here derive from the notion that the need to prevent unintended teenage pregnancy transcends affiliations of race, religion, politics, and socioeconomic status. Consequently, solutions to the problem require a strong commitment by diverse individuals and groups to work together. Although pregnancy is biologically determined, individuals and their communities can influence factors that surround it, particularly through programs that encourage the postponement of pregnancy and childbearing until parents are able to provide the necessities of life to their newborn. This book is designed to help communities bring together coalitions of policymakers, educators, health professionals, social service organizations, community groups, private businesses, parents, and teenagers in order to address the particular adolescent childbearing issues that have arisen in their area.

Section I begins with a brief overview of the nature of pregnancy and parenthood issues among teenagers in Chapter 1. Chapter 2 focuses on the need to address the problem through comprehensive prevention mechanisms, with an emphasis on two main strategies: (1) building the capacity to prevent teenage pregnancy through such efforts as education, communication, and counseling, and (2) enhancing the life options of teens by creating the opportunity structure to prevent high-risk behavior. Models for each of these two important strategies are described.

Because communities vary considerably in terms of their needs and circumstances, each must address the issue in ways that are appropriate to local conditions. This guidebook provides information that will allow individuals from diverse communities to select ideas and materials applicable to their own circumstances. Chapter 3 provides examples of local program models, broad-based coalitions, task forces, and state initiatives that provide important concepts for community leaders to consider as they begin to shape their own programs.

Section II outlines the details of how to develop a community-wide adolescent pregnancy prevention initiative. Chapter 4 describes how to bring together a coalition. This discussion is designed to assist individuals in a wide variety of communities that are at various stages of the planning process, and it provides detailed information about the structure of the coalition, who should be included, and how the group can resolve conflicts and take effective action. Chapter 5 discusses the all-important needs assessment, which enables a community group to determine the extent of the problem and evaluate available resources. This section also describes useful methods of data collection and provides detailed information about how to implement a workplan and construct a report. Also included is a guide to available sources that can help you to document the extent of the adolescent pregnancy problem within your community, the interventions and programs that are already in place to help meet the needs of this population, and information that can help you to identify gaps in existing services.

After the needs assessment is completed, program planning, implementation, and evaluation can be undertaken. Chapter 6 focuses on the utilization of needs assessment data to create an implementation plan that will be supported by a maximum number of community groups and individuals. A sample of a community-wide implementation plan is included along with a discussion of how to get such a plan adopted by the community at large. This is followed by a detailed discussion of implementation strategies in Chapter 7, including suggestions about how to strengthen collaborative relationships, how to initiate interagency activities, how to disseminate information, and how to develop new sources of funding. In Chapter 8 there is an outline of methods to evaluate the coalition's activities in order to determine the program's value — what is successful and what needs to be changed — and to assist in efforts to gain additional funding. It should also be noted that while this book is geared to the issue of adolescent pregnancy prevention, the planning process contained in Section II can also be applied to a variety of other pressing adolescent health and social issues, such as substance abuse or the school dropout problem.

SECTION I

A Profile of Teenage Pregnancy Prevention Programs

Chapter 1

A Conceptual Framework for Understanding Adolescent Pregnancy

Framing the Problem and the Solution

Teenage pregnancy was first recognized as a significant social and health problem almost two decades ago. At that time, it seemed that the best solution, if any solution was employed, was to provide young people with information through sex education classes, so they could make sound decisions about their sexuality; and (if they were sexually active) to give them access to contraceptive services. In light of our current understanding of the issue and increasing social pressures, we now know that these kinds of interventions are necessary but not sufficient.

Unlike other high-risk behaviors that threaten our young people's futures, pregnancy and parenthood are positively valued behaviors. The problems associated with early sexual activity, pregnancy, and parenthood are associated with the timing of those behaviors, not with the behaviors themselves. To persuade our youth that it is in their best interest to delay these behaviors, it is necessary to demonstrate that there are compelling opportunities in their present lives and their futures that will make the delay worthwhile.

Many disadvantaged teenagers are becoming parents because they realize they have only circumscribed access to social and economic opportunities. The point is not that large proportions of disadvantaged young people plan their pregnancies; it is that relatively small proportions take active and consistent measures to avoid pregnancy, and that when pregnancy occurs, disadvantaged adolescents are not likely to obtain abortions, to marry, or to put the child up for adoption. There is little reason to delay parenthood, it seems, in a life where expectations are already very low and skills are limited.

In order to prevent adolescent pregnancy, we must go beyond improvements in sex education and access to contraceptive services, and assist young people to make those major changes in their lives that will help them advance in school and prepare them to enter the labor force with the necessary skills. Many of the changes required are institutional: among other needs, schools have to be improved and employment opportunities broadened. Communities have to be stimulated to respond to the needs of their young people and families with a whole package of services. Our broadened perceptions of the problem also necessitate much greater involvement with males at every stage and in every intervention.

One way to conceptualize the strategies required to prevent adolescent pregnancy is to consider programs at two levels:

- Those interventions that will give young people the capacity to prevent pregnancy, including information that will help them make decisions concerning sexuality and access to contraceptive care.

- Those that will give young people the motivation and opportunity to continue in school and prepare for a productive life.

What Can We Learn From Research?

At the national level, we know a great deal about the sexual and reproductive behavior of young women. A series of studies beginning in 1971 has given us important insights into patterns of initiation of sexual intercourse, use of contraception, and the prevalence and consequences of teen pregnancy and childbearing. The National Academy of Sciences issued a two-volume report in 1987 that provides a compilation of research findings about adolescent pregnancy and parenting. The Children's Defense Fund, The Alan Guttmacher Institute, and the Center for Population Options all produce periodic reports of interest on this subject. The National Institute for Child Health and Human Development has supported many university-based researchers in studies of adolescent pregnancy. We will only touch on the highlights of these reports and studies here, but we encourage those who plan to develop community interventions to start with a firm base of knowledge about the issues. Specific resources are referenced at the end of this book.

The Reproductive Continuum

Adolescent pregnancy is the midpoint on a continuum of interconnected reproductive behaviors and decisions that stretch from the initiation of sexual activity through decisions about repeat births. One way to conceptualize issues relevant to adolescent pregnancy is to create a flow chart that starts with the teenage population and encompasses sexual involvement, contraceptive use, pregnancy, and births. (See Chart 1-1.)

Estimates of the magnitude of the problem and of the costs, complexity, degree of controversy, and probable success of intervention efforts are dependent upon which of the five main decision points is chosen as the primary focus of intervention. For

Chart 1-1
A Snapshot Profile of 15-19-Year-Old Teenage Women in 1985:
Sexual Activity, Pregnancy, Childbearing and Related Behaviors

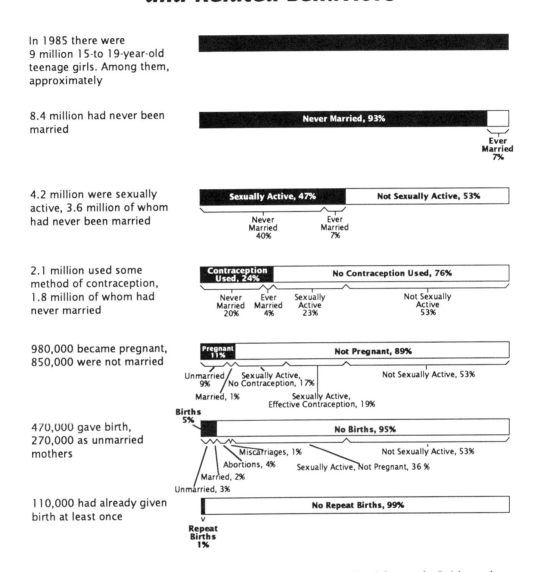

In 1985 there were 9 million 15-to 19-year-old teenage girls. Among them, approximately

8.4 million had never been married

4.2 million were sexually active, 3.6 million of whom had never been married

2.1 million used some method of contraception, 1.8 million of whom had never married

980,000 became pregnant, 850,000 were not married

470,000 gave birth, 270,000 as unmarried mothers

110,000 had already given birth at least once

Source: Children's Defense Fund, "Teenage Pregnancy: An Advocate's Guide to the Numbers," Washington, D.C.: Adolescent Pregnancy Prevention Clearinghouse, January/March, 1988.

example, if efforts concentrate on helping teens delay sexual activity, the primary target group is the 4.8 million teenage girls and 1.6 million teenage boys who are not yet sexually active. A large secondary target group includes the 10.5 million unmarried, sexually active teens (4.2 million of whom are girls) who might be successfully counseled to reconsider their sexual activity. There is approximately one sexually active teen for every teen who has not yet had intercourse. For every ten sexually active teenage girls, five did not use contraception, two became pregnant, and one gave birth.

You will probably find it difficult to reproduce this comprehensive information of the reproductive continuum for your community. While birth data are readily available, pregnancy data are often less accessible. Sexual activity data are estimates based on national surveys and are not available at the local level. Nonetheless, it is important to have this picture in mind as you consider approaches to addressing adolescent pregnancy in your community.

Breaking Down Teen Births into Categories

Another approach that will provide an important context for understanding adolescent pregnancy in your community includes the distribution of teen births broken down into categories reflecting age, race/ethnicity, and marital status. These essential data allow communities to determine what groups and strategies require their attention. For example, despite the fact that the media and others often portray teenage childbearing as a minority problem, the data show that two-thirds of these young mothers are white. Thus objective data challenge the myth that teenage pregnancy is solely a minority group problem. While racial and ethnic data vary among communities, one of the most important things you can do is assure that your community has the facts. (See Chart 1-2.)

Trends in Teenage Reproductive Behavior

Overall trends in teenage births and in unmarried teenage births are the products of distinct changes in behaviors along the reproductive continuum. Lack of uniformity among data sources prevents us from developing a clear picture of shifts in adolescent reproductive behavior over the last two decades. Nonetheless, a broad-brush view of rates of adolescent sexual activity, contraceptive use, abortion, birth, and marriage can be drawn.

- In varying degrees, rates of premarital sexual activity, contraceptive use, pregnancy, and abortion among teens rose during the 1970s and leveled off during the 1980s.

- Although sexual activity rates increased during the 1970s, teen birth rates declined, primarily because of wider use of contraceptives and abortion. Teen birth rates were essentially stable during the 1980s.

- The proportion of births to unmarried teens has increased sharply since 1970.

- Trends in the reportable sexually transmitted diseases (STD) gonorrhea and syphilis, reveal that teens aged 15 to 19 are at greatest risk. Among sexually active teens, the risk of STD is estimated to be two to three times higher than for individuals over 20.

- In 1986, among males aged 15 to 19, about 73,500 cases of gonorrhea and 1,800 cases of syphilis were reported. Among females aged 15 to 19, about 114,600 cases of gonorrhea and 2,500 cases of syphilis were reported in that year. An estimated

Chart 1-2

Births to Women Younger than 20
1985, by Race and Ethnicity, Marital Status, and Age

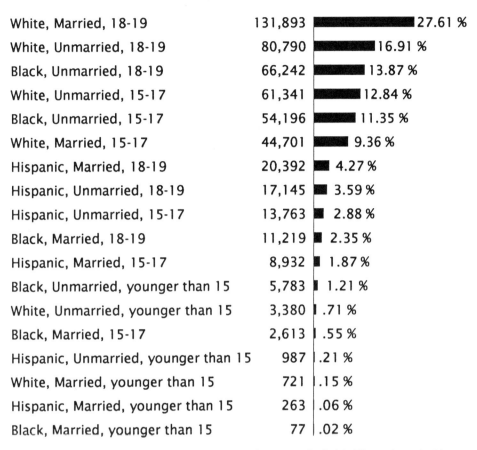

White, Married, 18-19	131,893	27.61 %
White, Unmarried, 18-19	80,790	16.91 %
Black, Unmarried, 18-19	66,242	13.87 %
White, Unmarried, 15-17	61,341	12.84 %
Black, Unmarried, 15-17	54,196	11.35 %
White, Married, 15-17	44,701	9.36 %
Hispanic, Married, 18-19	20,392	4.27 %
Hispanic, Unmarried, 18-19	17,145	3.59 %
Hispanic, Unmarried, 15-17	13,763	2.88 %
Black, Married, 18-19	11,219	2.35 %
Hispanic, Married, 15-17	8,932	1.87 %
Black, Unmarried, younger than 15	5,783	1.21 %
White, Unmarried, younger than 15	3,380	.71 %
Black, Married, 15-17	2,613	.55 %
Hispanic, Unmarried, younger than 15	987	.21 %
White, Married, younger than 15	721	.15 %
Hispanic, Married, younger than 15	263	.06 %
Black, Married, younger than 15	77	.02 %

Race Versus Ethnicity. The most important fact to remember when discussing racial and ethnic differences in sexual activity, preg-nancy, and childbearing is the difference between race and ethnicity. Hispanics are not a race but an ethnic group. Although there are dif-ferences in the preferred racial identification among the various subpopulations of Hispanics, in general about 95 percent of Hispanics who identify with a racial group identify themselves as white. In effect, this means in any table giving racial and ethnic data, the numbers of white, black and Hispanic teens will add up to more than the total because some Hispanics are counted in both the Hispanic and white or black columns. There is no simple way to correct for this double counting.

Source: Children's Defense Fund, "Teenage Pregnancy: An Advocate's Guide to the Numbers," Washington, D.C.: Adolescent Pregnancy Prevention Clearinghouse, January/March, 1988.

one million teens suffer from chlamydia infections each year. Nearly 900 young people aged 13 to 21 have diagnosed cases of AIDS, and the number of HIV-infected teens is as yet undocumented.

Targeting the Boys

In recent years, as both the consequences of early parenthood and the number of single teen mothers have increased, there has been greater interest in reproductive behavior of adolescent males and in their response to early parenthood. The teenage male's role and attitude have been neglected. There is a growing consensus that, to be effective, adolescent pregnancy prevention strategies must target boys as well as girls. Unfortunately, current interest far outstrips available information. What we do know, however, is sufficient to confirm certain assumptions about boys and to dispel others:

- At every age, young men are less likely to be married than young women. In 1984, 13 percent of all 18- and 19-year-old girls, but only 3 percent of 18- and 19-year-old boys, had ever married.

- At every age, adolescent boys are more likely to report being sexually active than are adolescent girls. Almost 65 percent of all boys, compared to 44 percent of all girls, report having initiated sex before age 18.

- Boys are somewhat less likely than girls to report having used some form of contraception at first intercourse, but the differences are not great – 44 percent of boys versus 49 percent of girls.

- There are no reliable data on the number of teenage boys who have fathered a baby. Data from birth certificates, however, suggest that most fathers of the children of teen mothers are not teens themselves. Fewer than two-thirds of teen mothers provide information about the father on the birth certificate, but of those who do, over half report that the father is over 20. It is estimated that the fathers are generally about two years older than the mother.

Predictors of Early Sexual Activity, Contraceptive Use, Pregnancy, and Parenthood

By carefully examining basic data on adolescents who are sexually active and at risk of unintended pregnancy, we can gain an understanding of trends in these behaviors and the magnitude of the problem. Through this information researchers have compiled a theoretical framework on which to base recommendations for policy and programmatic changes. The factors associated with early sexual activity, contraceptive use, pregnancy, and parenthood fall into four broad categories – age, race/ethnicity, individual characteristics and behaviors, and family background.

- *Age.* Younger teens who are sexually active are less likely than older teens to use contraceptives, which places them at a heightened risk of pregnancy.

- *Race/ethnicity.* Although white teens account for approximately two-thirds of teen births, black and Hispanic teens are disproportionately likely to be teen parents, and blacks are disproportionately likely to be *single* teen parents. Black teen birth rates are more than twice as high as those for whites, as are those for Hispanics. Birth rates among unmarried black teens are more than four times higher than those for unmarried whites. The racial differences in sexual activity and contraceptive use are not as striking, but they do exist, and reported rates of sexual activity among young black males are very high compared to those of whites.

- *Individual behavior.* Not surprisingly, girls who become teen mothers are more likely than those who delay pregnancy and parenthood to have less knowledge of the risk of pregnancy as a result of sexual intercourse, and to be poorer contraceptive users. Teen mothers and fathers are also found to have poorer academic skills. Those with reading and math skills that place them in the bottom fifth of their peer group are three times as likely to be teen parents as those with average academic skills. Additionally, girls who drop out of school are more likely to be at risk of early pregnancy. A national sample of 19- to 23-year-old women shows that among those with the lowest basic educational skills, 61 percent are mothers and 30 percent have two or more children. In the top group with high basic skills, the comparable figures are 7 percent and 2 percent. Research also indicates that young women who terminate their pregnancies with abortions are different from those who continue their pregnancies; like those who delay pregnancy, these young women are more likely to be doing well in school and to have high educational and occupational expectations.

- *Family and community background.* Teens from poor families and from single-parent families, and those who live in poor neighborhoods and/or attend all-minority segregated schools are more likely to be teen mothers.

These categories of variables above are interrelated – minority youths are most likely to be poor, to come from single-parent families, to attend poor quality and segregated schools, and to have weak academic skills and little attachment to school. Research has shown that once racial and ethnic differences in family income and academic skills are taken into account, minority teens are no more likely to be mothers than are white teens. Black, white, or Hispanic, 20 percent of 16- to 19-year-old young women who come from families with below-poverty incomes and who have poor academic skills are mothers, compared to between 3 and 5 percent of teens of the same race or ethnicity who have solid academic skills and whose families have above-poverty incomes. No significant differences in the probability of childbearing remain after accounting for basic academic skills and poverty.

Research findings produce broad generalizations, identifying specific characteristics that correlate with higher risk of sexual activity, pregnancy, or parenthood. Obviously, every teenage mother does not come from a poor family, and every young woman who has an abortion is not a high achiever. Even in the highest risk groups, ample numbers of young people are not sexually active, not pregnant, not parents, and not unmarried parents. This demonstrates that effective strategies for lowering pregnancy rates among every group can be developed. It would also be useful to study these exceptions to discover what personal and environmental factors contribute to their successful decision-making and avoidance of pregnancy. This information would also help guide us to successful intervention.

Related Problem Behaviors

Much attention is given to the concept of a problem behavior syndrome, that is, placing early sexual intercourse along with early smoking and drinking, drug use, and delinquency as behaviors that have a high probability of occurring simultaneously. Research lends evidence to this grouping; one study associates early sexual activity with early drug use, and another relates it to delinquency. Researchers report a higher teen pregnancy rate among users of illicit drugs. Low socioeconomic status, as measured by parent's income and educational level, is clearly a factor in school failure and delinquency, as well as in teen pregnancy. The data on substance abuse are less clear.

It is possible to distinguish between responsible and irresponsible sexual behavior, just as we differentiate between experimenting with substances and becoming an alcoholic or an addict. Adolescents have a clear developmental need for new experiences. Our attention here is focused only on those interrelated high-risk behaviors that lead to negative consequences for the child, family, community, and society. There appear to be six common determinants that predict high-risk behaviors such as early childbearing, substance abuse, delinquency, and school failure:

1. Low school achievement

2. Lack of parental support

3. Lack of resistance to peer influences

4. Nonconformity/rebelliousness

5. Early initiation of any of the high-risk behaviors

6. Residence in a disadvantaged neighborhood

Providing Teens with the Capacity to Prevent Pregnancy

Sexuality and Family Life Education

The initial step toward providing the capacity to prevent pregnancy requires two critical components: sexuality and family life education, and contraceptive services. To be effective, these latter services must also provide counseling and assistance in avoiding sexually transmitted disease and accessing abortion services.

Most communities already have some sort of family life education program in place. A recent survey by The Alan Guttmacher Institute indicates that 80 percent of all states either mandate or encourage the teaching of sex education in the public schools; 90 percent of large school districts support such instruction. Timely access to this information is critical to any pregnancy prevention effort. Young people need to know how to make responsible decisions and how to interact with peers, parents, teachers, and others in implementing these decisions. Decisions about sexual activity, contraceptive use and pregnancy are most dangerous when they are made in the absence of accurate information and honest discussion. Yet information alone is not enough to change behavior. Communities must look for ways not only to expand access to existing family life education, but also to incorporate new approaches such as social skills training, group discussion with boys and girls, broader instruction in life planning, small group and individual counseling, and social modeling opportunities.

Family life education should be offered in settings and formats that appeal to boys as well as girls.

Contraceptive Services

A 1987 National Academy of Sciences report concluded that "the major strategy for reducing early unintended pregnancy must be the encouragement of diligent contraceptive use by all sexually active teenagers," males as well as females. Most communities have family planning clinics that serve many of their adolescents. These services can be upgraded with more individual counseling, outreach, follow-up, and other innovative approaches. Family planning agencies can be brought into closer collaboration with other youth-serving agencies and schools. Birth control services can be offered in many different settings, including clinics in or adjacent to schools, and comprehensive community health and recreation agencies. Condoms can be widely distributed through youth outreach workers in recreation and sports centers and clubs, gas stations, and other community-based locations.

A Word of Caution

No matter how carefully your pregnancy prevention project is crafted and presented, it is likely that you will have to address two controversial issues: abortion and AIDS. Both have such obvious connections to the broader issue of adolescent sexual activity that you cannot expect to avoid them, and should plan carefully how they will be handled. We suggest that, with advance planning, these issues can not only be addressed but also used in developing and promoting a pregnancy prevention strategy for your community.

Sexually Transmitted Disease Services

Pregnancy is not the only consequence of unprotected sexual activity, and it is no longer the most serious. Early initiation of sex and frequent sex with multiple sexual partners results in high rates of sexually transmitted diseases (STDs) that have serious and sometimes fatal health consequences. Rising rates of gonorrhea, chlamydia and herpes among young people have been shown to lead to rising incidences of pelvic inflammatory disease (PID), infertility, ectopic pregnancies, cervical cancer, and infections in the infant. The Acquired Immune Deficiency Syndrome (AIDS) epidemic presents new challenges. Although the long incubation period associated with AIDS means that few adolescents have yet been identified with the disease, many have lifestyles that incorporate behavior that increases their risk of infection, including multiple sexual partners, sex with older partners, unprotected sexual activity, and intravenous drug use.

The threat of AIDS has led to the development of a much more aggressive and straightforward presentation of sexual information and services to children and youth. These programs can be used to expand pregnancy prevention efforts in communities.

However, efforts are necessary to ensure that AIDS education and services do not take the place of broad, comprehensive family life and decision-making education and, similarly, that condom distribution programs do not diminish efforts to make comprehensive reproductive health counseling and services available.

Abortion Services

Although the subject of abortion is difficult in every community, the current reality is that teenagers use abortion to prevent unwanted childbearing. A comprehensive strategy to ameliorate the consequences of early pregnancy should address the need among teenagers for safe and accessible abortions. If a well functioning prevention strategy were in place, however, the need for abortion would be dramatically reduced.

Creating the Opportunity Structure to Prevent Pregnancy

Changing the setting in which young people grow and learn is a much more complex task than ensuring capacity to prevent pregnancy. Nevertheless, disadvantaged children cannot adequately utilize the services outlined above unless they have both the basic skills required and the sense that their lives will change if they delay early childbearing. Altering the learning and living environment implies more than courses in self-esteem or motivational efforts. There are three general areas of intervention: education, employment, and social support.

Enhanced Education

All children are entitled to a quality education that produces an acceptable level of literacy and certain basic skills. In many communities, school failure is rampant and dropout rates are excessive. Early childhood education can have a significant impact on later achievement, as well as on rates of pregnancy. In some communities, the whole educational system may require reorganization. In other communities, alternative educational interventions can be offered to high-risk children. Young people who have already dropped out can be encouraged to continue their education through school or community-based efforts.

Employment Potential

It has been estimated that 25 percent of our current youth population will not be able to hold jobs in the future unless intensive remediation takes place. The career ladder is established early in life. In order to move up the ladder, children must understand that certain levels of achievement are necessary for certain jobs. Beginning in the elementary grades, they can be exposed to a wide array of jobs and careers, and through school and community service experiences they can begin to build the skills and attitudes sought by employers. As they reach their late teens, young people can be helped to apply for jobs and maintain employment in placements that increase their skills. The business community can be involved in collaborative efforts to create employment opportunities, including "job shadowing," mentor programs, and apprenticeships.

Social Support

Many disadvantaged children lack sustained, effective support from parents, peers, and neighbors, who may themselves be at high risk of problem behaviors. Parent education programs can be effective in informing parents about programs designed to serve their children and in assisting them to develop supportive behavior. The solution goes far beyond parental involvement, however. In many communities there is a basic lack of social as well as basic financial support. Few coordinated programs and services for disadvantaged youths and families exist. Clearly, these high-risk adolescents are most successful when family, community, and public institutions work toward common goals. Community-wide mechanisms can be developed that insure that every high-risk child is connected to responsible adults who can track and monitor what goes on in the child's life. Community-based after-school programs, community service efforts, even incentive programs that offer students rewards for positive behaviors (staying in school, avoiding pregnancy) can all be components of a system of support services.

Key Factors in Successful Programs

Although much is yet to be learned and documented about adolescent pregnancy and treatment programs, the following have been identified as key factors in successful programs (Brindis and Jeremy, 1988):

- *Early Intervention:* Whether the goal is abstinence, effective use of contraception, appropriate prenatal care, or improved maternal and child health, the earlier the medical, psychosocial, nutritional, or educational interventions are introduced, the higher the likelihood of successful outcomes.

- *Accessibility and Acceptability:* Programs and services need to be physically accessible (on major bus lines, close to a targeted neighborhood, near or on a school campus), affordable (inexpensive, sliding scale fee, or free), culturally sensitive (with multilingual and multiethnic male or female staff, as appropriate), and psychologically acceptable to the user.

- *Continuity:* Programs with long-term follow-up and continued tracking are the most successful. The needs of adolescents, especially in the high-risk, low-income groups, are so extensive that without sustained social and financial support, maintaining progress is difficult.

- *Targeting:* Teenagers' needs differ by age group, gender, and socioeconomic and cultural background. Appropriate services sensitive to the needs of the particular target group increase effectiveness.

- *Institutionalization:* Without a commitment from school districts, medical care providers, parents, community groups, government, and private agencies to integrate prevention and treatment strategies into ongoing efforts, programs are often financially fragile and of limited long-range impact.

The key participants in these successful programs have been the following:

- *Families, nuclear and extended:* Studies have demonstrated repeatedly the importance of family values and support. Family communication, especially between mother and daughter, can lower the rate of adolescent sexual activity. If a teenager gives birth and decides to raise the baby, family support – emotional, financial, and/or childcare – can reduce the likelihood of negative consequences.

- *Schools:* Teachers, guidance counselors, nurses, and support staff in schools play an important role in pregnancy postponement by helping teenagers continue their educations, develop their decision-making skills, and expand their employment opportunities and life options. Schools also provide a setting in which family life education can be integrated into activities and other subject matter.

- *Community-based organizations:* This category includes ethnic, cultural, and religious organizations, privately and publicly funded not-for-profit agencies, and public social service agencies. Through their wide range of services, they can reach teenagers who have dropped out of school or graduated, as well as those still in school.

Summary

There are many different ways to view the problem of adolescent pregnancy. How one defines the problem is closely related to how one defines the solution. It would be a lot easier if we as a society could "just say no" and young people would behave accordingly. We suggest that the problem is more complex than that, and no one solution will suffice. Many institutions are implicated: the health system, the educational system, business, the media, and of course, the family. We propose that teen pregnancy be viewed as a symptom of the epidemic of high-risk behavior that is severely limiting the potential of American youth. We have shown how these behaviors are interrelated and how they occur inequitably among disadvantaged families. This understanding of the holistic nature of the problem suggests that the solutions must be interrelated as well. A 1987 National Academy of Sciences report contained some excellent advice about this issue:

"The hope for a solution to the problem of teenage pregnancy is illusory without simultaneous amelioration of some of these contributing factors. Pending such comprehensive change, the panel urges prevention rather than denial, kindness rather than exhortation, and research rather than doctrine."

Appendix 1-1

Adolescent Pregnancy and Parenting Fact Sheet

---

*T*his fact sheet and the following references are a compilation of a number of worksheets developed for the Adolescent Pregnancy Subcommittee of the March of Dimes' Healthy Mothers/Healthy Babies Coalition by the following national organizations: The Alan Guttmacher Institute, The Children's Defense Fund, the National Organization on Adolescent Pregnancy and Parenting, Inc., and the Center for Population Options. For additional information, refer to the General Resource Directory on page 261 for addresses and phone numbers.

U.S. Teen Births in 1986

- In 1986, there were 472,081 births to teenagers (younger than 20 years old). This represents about one birth for every 20 teenage girls between the ages of 15 and 19. Teen births accounted for 12.6 percent of the births to all women in 1986. (1)

- Two-thirds (315,335) of the births to teens in 1986 were to white teens, and slightly less than one-third (141,606) were to black teens. Fourteen percent (63,816 births) were to Hispanic teens. (Note: Hispanics are an ethnic group, not a race, and therefore the white, black and Hispanic percentages will not sum to the total for all races.) Minority teens, however, are disproportionately likely to give birth. In 1986, for example, there were 41.8 births for every 1000 white teens ages 15-19, and 98.1 births for every 1000 black teens. (2)

- About 40 percent of the nearly one million teen pregnancies each year end in abortion, with the remainder resulting in live births and miscarriages. Young teenagers are more likely than older teenagers to terminate a pregnancy by abortion but, at all ages, teens are more likely to carry a pregnancy to term than to terminate it. (3)

Trends in Teen Birth Rates and Marital Status

- After generally declining or remaining stable during the late 1970s and early 1980s, the birth rate of very young teens (ages 10 to 14) began to rise in 1984. In 1986, it rose to 1.3 births per 1000, the highest level since 1975. All of this increase is due to a rise in the birth rate of very young nonwhite teens. The birth rates of very young white teens have been fairly stable. (4)

- While minority teens are disproportionately likely to be unmarried at the time of birth, the increase in the proportion of teen births that are to unmarried teens is found among all teens — white, black, or Hispanic. By 1986, 49 percent of the white, 55 percent of the Hispanic, and 90 percent of the black teens were unmarried when their child was born. (5)

Consequences of Teen Parenting

School

- Teen girls with poor basic skills are five times as likely to become mothers before age 16 as are those with average basic skills. (6)

- Annually, at least 40,000 teen girls drop out of school because of pregnancy. (7)

- Nearly 65 percent of young mothers under 14 and 50 percent of those 15-19 years old do not complete high school. (8)

- The more years of schooling that a young woman has completed, the more likely she is to delay childbearing. (9)

- Research on school age mothers' educational patterns indicates that they are more likely to complete high school (and delay subsequent pregnancies) if they are enrolled in school during pregnancy and after birth. (10)

- 18 and 19 year old males with poor basic academic skills are three times as likely to become teen fathers as those with average basic academic skills. (11)

Health

- The maternal mortality rate for mothers under 15 is 60 percent greater than for women in their 20s. (12)

- Only 53.5 percent of teenage women get prenatal care in the first trimester, compared to 76.2 percent of all women. In addition, 12.2 percent of teenage women get late or no prenatal care, compared with only 5.7 percent of all women. (13)

- There are 18 deaths for every 1000 births to mothers under 17; the rate for mothers in their 20s is 10.3 per 1000. (14)

Economic

- Women who enter parenthood as teenagers are at greater risk of living in poverty, both in the short and long term. (15)

- Because a teen parent lacks job skills and work experience, she earns half the lifetime earnings of a woman who waits until 20 to have her first child. (16)

- In 1987 alone, the U.S. spent $19.27 billion on Aid for Families with Dependent Children (AFDC), Medicaid, and Food Stamp payments to families begun when the mother was a teenager. (17)

- Fifty-three percent of AFDC payments go to support families begun when the mother was a teenager. (18)

- Only 14% of unmarried mothers receive child support from the fathers. (19)

Public Opinion on Sex Education

- According to a variety of public opinion polls, more than 85 percent of the American public supports sex education in the schools. This support has been increasing steadily in recent years. (20)

- According to the Yankelovich et al. poll, most Americans believe that students who take sex education courses in school are less likely to become (or get someone) pregnant, more likely to practice birth control when they have sex and less likely to get a sexually transmitted disease. Forty-three percent think students will be less likely to engage in sex at an earlier age, while 24 percent think they will be more likely to do so. (21)

Impact of Sex Education

- Study after study has shown that sex education is effective in increasing young people's knowledge. Indeed, the 1986 Harris poll found that teens who had had "comprehensive" sex education were twice as likely as those who had no sex education to have accurate information related to the risk of pregnancy. Available evidence indicates that students do not develop more permissive attitudes toward sexual activity as a result of sex education. Sex education does not appear to either encourage or discourage teenagers from becoming sexually active, but several studies have shown better contraceptive use among sexually active teens who have had instruction. (22-27)

The Role of the Family

- Eighty-four percent of adults with children aged 11-18 said, in a public opinion poll, that they have talked with their child about sex and pregnancy, but only 62 percent had discussed the use of contraception. A poll of teenagers aged 12-17 found that 68 percent reported having talked with their parents about sex and how pregnancy is caused; but only half of these had conversations that addressed birth control. (28)

- A study of teenagers attending family planning clinics found that if their parents had to be notified, 23 percent said they would stop coming; 12 percent would switch to less effective non-prescription methods, 4 percent would try rhythm or withdrawal and 5 percent would use no contraception. Only 2 percent said they would refrain from sexual relations. This indicates that the effect of a parental consent or notification requirement would likely be an upswing in unintended pregnancies. (29)

Characteristics of Adolescents' Contraceptive Use

• Eighty-five percent of sexually active women aged 15-19 have used contraception at some time, but 37 percent use a method only sometimes and 15 percent never use a method. Only 48 percent of teenagers use contraception at first intercourse. (30)

• Seventy-three percent of teenage women who go to a clinic or a physician seeking effective contraception are already sexually active, and usually they have been so for about a year. (31)

• Within two years, nearly 50 percent of teenagers who use no contraception become pregnant, while 25 percent of those who use a nonmedical method and only 15 percent of those who use a medical method do so. (32)

• Nearly 4 million teenage women are sexually active and in need of contraception to avoid unintended pregnancy. (33)

• The leading reason given by teenagers who have intercourse and usually do not use birth control is that they had not expected to have sex (21%). Other frequently cited reasons are that they do not want to use it, do not want to take the time, or they think they won't get pregnant (9% each). (34)

• Sexually active teenagers in the U.S. are less likely to use contraception than those in Britain, Canada, Sweden or the Netherlands. They are also less likely to use the most effective method, the pill. (35)

• The younger the couple, the less likely they are to use contraception, but if they do use contraception, male methods (condoms and withdrawal) are the more likely. Two out of five teen women who used contraception during their most recent intercourse reported that they used male contraceptive methods. (36)

• More than a quarter of school-age women who get abortions have never used contraception. Those that do use a method often use one of the less effective ones, such as the condom or withdrawal. Condoms are an effective method for decreasing the transmission of sexually transmitted diseases. Used without foam, condoms have a user effectiveness of 97% in preventing pregnancy, while used together with foam, effectiveness increases to 99%. (37)

• Society's double standard of acceptable sexual behavior sends mixed signals to teens. Girls are more likely than boys to have motivation to use and knowledge about contraception. But they are unlikely to have contraceptives available when intercourse might occur because the double standard signals that it's wrong for girls to have, or plan to have, sex. (38)

- Boys know less than girls do about contraception and pregnancy risk, and are more likely to be misinformed. Unfortunately, the popular misconception that boys are unwilling to listen to information about sexuality and contraception limits adults' efforts to talk with boys. (39)

Abortion

- Since abortion became legal nationwide in 1973, over 5 million teenage women (plus many older women) have terminated unintended pregnancies by abortion. Legal abortion was, in large part, responsible for the decline in the teen birthrate during the early 1970s. (40)

- Of the 1.6 million abortions obtained by U.S. women in 1986, an estimated 26 percent were by teenagers. The rate of teen abortions, or the number per 1,000 teenage women, has remained relatively stable throughout the late 1970s and early 1980s. (41, 42, 43)

- Legal abortion is far safer than childbirth. Among women of all ages, the risk of death associated with childbirth is roughly ten times as high as that associated with abortion. (Less than one woman of 100,000 who obtain an abortion dies.) Among teens, the risk of abortion relative to childbirth is even lower, both because they are less likely than older women to die following an abortion and because the risks associated with pregnancy and childbirth are greater for very young women. (44, 45, 46)

References

1. Children's Defense Fund, "Teen Births: Snapshot and Trends," Healthy Mothers, Healthy Babies Coalition, Nov. 1988.

2. Children's Defense Fund, "Teen Births: Snapshot and Trends," Healthy Mothers, Healthy Babies Coalition, Nov. 1988.

3. S.K. Henshaw, "Characteristics of U.S. Women Having Abortions, 1982-1983," *Family Planning Perspectives*, 19:5, 1987.

4. Children's Defense Fund, "Teen Births: Snapshot and Trends," Healthy Mothers, Healthy Babies Coalition, Nov. 1988.

5. Children's Defense Fund, "Teen Births: Snapshot and Trends," Healthy Mothers, Healthy Babies Coalition, Nov. 1988.

6. National Organization on Adolescent Pregnancy and Parenting, Inc., "Educational Consequences of Teen Parenthood."

7. National Organization on Adolescent Pregnancy and Parenting, Inc., "Educational Consequences of Teen Parenthood."

8. National Organization on Adolescent Pregnancy and Parenting, Inc., "Educational Consequences of Teen Parenthood."

9. National Organization on Adolescent Pregnancy and Parenting, Inc., "Educational Consequences of Teen Parenthood."

10. National Organization on Adolescent Pregnancy and Parenting, Inc., "Educational Consequences of Teen Parenthood."

11. National Organization on Adolescent Pregnancy and Parenting, Inc., "Educational Consequences of Teen Parenthood."

12. The National Commission to Prevent Infant Mortality, *Death Before Life: The Tragedy of Infant Mortality;* Appendix, August, 1988, p. 103.

13. Children's Defense Fund, *The Health of America's Children*, 1988, p. 29.

14. The National Commission to Prevent Infant Mortality, *Death Before Life: The Tragedy of Infant Mortality;* Appendix, August, 1988, p. 103.

15. National Organization on Adolescent Pregnancy and Parenting, Inc., "Employment Consequences of Teen Parenting."

16. National Organization on Adolescent Pregnancy and Parenting, Inc., "Employment Consequences of Teen Parenting."

17. Center for Population Options, *1988 Report: Estimates of Public Cost for Teenage Childbearing in 1987, 1988.*

18. M.R. Burt, *Estimates of Public Costs for Teenage Childbearing*, Center for Population Options, 1986.

19. H.J. Nicholson, "Teenage Pregnancy: Prevention is Critical," *Youth Policy*, 10(5): 26, May 1988.

20. Louis Harris and Associates, Inc., "Public Attitudes Toward Teenage Pregnancy, Sex Education and Birth Control," New York, New York, 1988, p. 24; and Louis Harris and Associates, Inc., "Public Attitudes About Sex Education, Family Planning and Abortion in the United States," New York, New York, 1985, p. 44.

21. Memorandum to All Data Users from Hal Quinley, Senior Associate, Yankelovich, Clancy Shulman on Time/Yankelovich, Clancy, Shulman Poll Findings on Sex Education, dated Nov. 17, 1986, Table 4.

22. A.M. Kenney, M.T. Orr, "Sex Education: An Overview of Current Programs, Policies and Research," *Phi Delta Kappan*, 65:491, 1984.

23. Louis Harris and Associates, Inc., "American Teenagers Speak: Sex, Myths, T.V. and Birth Control," New York, New York, 1986, p. 33.

24. D.A. Dawson, "The Effects of Sex Education on Adolescent Behavior," *Family Planning Perspectives*, 18:162, 1986.

25. M.D. Benson, C. Perlman, J.J. Sciarra, "Sex Education in the Inner City: Learning and Retention," *Journal of the American Medical Association*, 255:43, 1986.

26. W. Marsiglio, F.L. Mott, "The Impact of Sex Education on Sexual Activity, Contraceptive Use and Premarital Pregnancy Among American Teenagers," *Family Planning Perspectives, 18:151, 1986.*

27. M. Zelnik, Y.J. Kim, "Sex Education and Its Association with Teenage Sexual Activity, Pregnancy and Contraceptive Use," *Family Planning Perspectives*, 14:117, 1982.

28. Louis Harris and Associates, Inc., "Public Attitudes Toward Teenage Pregnancy, Sex Education and Birth Control, " New York, New York, 1988, p. 20; and Louis Harris and Associates, Inc., "American Teenagers Speak: Sex, Myths, T.V. and Birth Control," New York, New York, 1986, p. 7.

29. A.M. Kenney, J.D. Forrest, A. Torres, "Storm Over Washington: The Parental Notification Proposal," *Family Planning Perspectives*, 14:185, 1982.

30. *Risking the Future, Adolescent Sexuality, Pregnancy and Childbearing,* National Research Council, National Academy Press: Washington, D.C., 1987, p. 46-47, Table 2-8.

31. M. Zelnik, M.A. Koenig, Y.J. Kim, "Sources of Prescription Contraceptives and Subsequent Pregnancy Among Young Women," *Family Planning Perspectives,* 16:6, 1984.

32. *Risking the Future, Adolescent Sexuality, Pregnancy and Childbearing,* National Research Council, National Academy Press: Washington, D.C., 1987, p. 49.

33. *Risking the Future, Adolescent Sexuality, Pregnancy and Childbearing,* National Research Council, National Academy Press: Washington, D.C., 1987, p. 73, Fig. 2-5.

34. Louis Harris and Associates, Inc., "American Teenagers Speak: Sex, Myths, T.V. and Birth Control," New York, New York, 1986, p. 28.

35. E.F. Jones, J.D. Forrest, N. Goldman, S.K. Henshaw, R. Lincoln, J.I. Rosoff, C.F. Westoff, D. Wolf, "Teenage Pregnancy in Developed Countries: Determinants and Policy Implications," *Family Planning Perspectives*, 17:53, 1985.

36. Children's Defense Fund, "What About the Boys? Teenage Pregnancy and Parenthood," Healthy Mothers, Healthy Babies Coalition, November 1988.

37. S.K. Henshaw and J. Silverman, "The Characteristics and Prior Contraceptive Use of U.S. Abortion Patients," *Family Planning Perspectives*, 20:158, 1988.

38. Children's Defense Fund, "What About the Boys? Teenage Pregnancy and Parenthood," Healthy Mothers, Healthy Babies Coalition, November 1988.

39. Children's Defense Fund, "What About the Boys? Teenage Pregnancy and Parenthood," Healthy Mothers, Healthy Babies Coalition, November 1988.

40. The Alan Guttmacher Institute (AGI), unpublished data.

41. S.K. Henshaw, J.D. Forrest, J. Van Vort, "Abortion Services in the United States, 1984 and 1985," *Family Planning Perspectives*, 19:63, 1987.

42. S.K. Henshaw and J. Silverman, "The Characteristics and Prior Contraceptive Use of U.S. Abortion Patients," *Family Planning Perspectives*, 20:158, 1988.

43. S.K. Henshaw and J. Van Vort, eds., *Abortion Services in the United States, Each State and Metropolitan Area, 1984-1985*, New York: AGI, 1988.

44. C. Tietze, S.K. Henshaw, "Induced Abortion: A World Review, 1986," New York: AGI, 1986.

45. H.K. Antrash et al., "Legal Abortion Mortality in the United States: 1972 - 1982," *American Journal of Obstetrics and Gynecology*, 156:605, March 1987.

46. AGI, "Teenage Pregnancy: The Problem That Hasn't Gone Away," New York, New York, 1981.

Chapter 2

Preventing Teenage Pregnancy: Creating the Capacity and the Opportunity Structure

*T*he argument that teens need both the capacity and the opportunity structure to delay pregnancy suggests that solutions to the teenage pregnancy problem extend far beyond the boundaries of traditional strategies – sexuality-specific education, counseling, and contraceptive information and services. However, any program designed to delay adolescent childbearing will be inadequate without inclusion of these educational and informational tools and ready accessibility to contraceptive services. All young people today must come to understand the risks and consequences of sexual activity and pregnancy in order to make responsible choices and to take seriously their decisions about sexual activity. The teen who has access to timely comprehensive sexuality-specific information and services is more likely to delay pregnancy than one who does not.

There is no need for each community to design a new program in the field of adolescent pregnancy, since so many excellent programs have already been developed, tested and made available for general use. Later in this chapter we will describe some examples. First, however, here is a brief discussion on the different needs of teenagers with and without solid life options.

The presence or absence of life opportunities is generally considered to be the most critical factor in adolescent childbearing. The teen who is doing well in school and in the family and community is more likely to delay pregnancy than the one who is not. Research reviewed by the National Academy of Sciences also suggests that teens' decisions about sexual activity and contraception are tied closely to their aspirations and to their perceptions of the opportunities open to them (Hayes, 1987). Teens with strong achievement orientations and clear goals for the future, therefore, are likely, if sexually active, to be regular and effective contraceptive users. In contrast, young people facing limited life options – poor teens and teens with few academic skills – are at greatest risk for early parenthood, whether or not sexually specific services are available to them. Ready access to family planning services is needed for both groups of young people.

Millions of young women who truncate their educations by leaving high school to bear children fail to consider actively other options because they *generally do not see better alternatives*. Before they reach adolescence, the force motivating them to improve their lives has often been damaged.

Doing well in school is as important as staying in school. Poor basic academic skills influence life options and the transition to adulthood in direct and indirect ways. Students with serious basic skill deficiencies often have encountered failure so frequently that their self-esteem in nonacademic areas also lags behind that of their peers. It is this combination of limited opportunities and a less developed sense of their own potential that places poor and minority youths at particularly high risk of early parenthood.

Teens for whom the basic supports are in place (the educational, occupational and family experiences, and opportunities that give them compelling reasons to want to delay parenthood) may only need comprehensive sex education and access to contra-ceptive counseling and services. Teens for whom these basic supports are weak, however, may need a combination of sexuality-specific information, counseling, and supportive programs and services that help them and their families to broaden their experiences, sharpen their expectations, and increase their access to and utilization of education, employment opportunities, health care, family support, and recreation.

In summary:

• All teens need sex education.

• Sexually active teens need contraceptive services and counseling.

• At-risk teens (those not doing well in school, not connected to community institu-tions, etc.) need a cadre of support services that allow them to identify and take maximum advantage of the opportunities available.

• Communities and institutions serving at-risk youth need to increase the quality, availability, and accessibility of the services they offer teens.

The first two categories are traditionally defined as the domain of those interested in pregnancy prevention – *"capacity building."* The second two categories fall under the

umbrella term – *"improving life options."* We make distinctions between supportive
services that can help youths take advantage of opportunities available to them
(tutoring and after-school programs, recreation, counseling, health and mental health
services) and major reforms that increase the opportunities available (educational
reform, efforts to increase the minimum wage, youth employment). The third category
– supportive services – will be important to those interested in developing strategies
for high-risk youth. Those interested in pregnancy prevention would be wise to
become active in efforts in the community to improve schools, youth employment
opportunities, etc. However, these very major reforms are not viable components of a
pregnancy prevention agenda *independent* of efforts to make family life and contraception services more readily available to teenagers.

Building the Capacity to Prevent Teenage Pregnancy

Information and Counseling

Sex education programs – also referred to as family life education, health education,
health promotion, human development, family living, and a host of other terms – have
been one of the more controversial responses to the teenage pregnancy problem.
Proponents argue that better family life/sex education efforts will help reduce the
alarming incidence of teenage pregnancy, that too few institutions offer appropriate
instruction, and that those that do, offer too little too late. Opponents charge that sex
education actually may fuel the problem by encouraging teenage sexual activity,
although a number of research studies refute this position (Kirby 1984, Dawson 1986,
Marsiglio and Mott 1986). There is neither empirical evidence that sex education
increases teen pregnancy rates, nor evidence that sex education reduces teen pregnancy rates (Marsiglio and Mott, 1986; Dawson, 1986; Zelnik and Kim, 1982; Louis
Harris and Associates, 1986). A challenge to family life educators has been the fact
that while most of the existing programs appear to positively affect 1) knowledge,
particularly for younger adolescents in topics of birth control, sexually transmitted
diseases, and the probability of becoming pregnant; 2) skills, so that students show
improvements in communication and decision-making skills; and 3) parent-child
communication, resulting in a greater sense of comfort in discussing sexual issues
within the family, family life programs have not been shown to affect behavior. Given
that these interventions are short-term in the full life span of the adolescent, are often
diluted, and come much too late in students' educational experience, these results are
not surprising. Research indicates, however, that sexuality-specific information and
services may increase sexual responsibility and contraceptive use among sexually
active teens. One study, in fact, found that sexually active teenage females who have
had sex education are less likely to become pregnant than their counterparts who
have had no such instruction (Zelnik and Kim, 1982).

The idea of sex education, especially in the schools, has been around since the turn of
the century, with the original goal of teaching sexual restraint. Traditional sex education has been confined to highly structured sessions covering a limited range of
topics. Family life/sex education encompasses a great deal more.

The goals of family life/sex education can be divided into three broad categories:

- To increase knowledge about anatomy and physiology, sexuality, sexually transmitted diseases, pregnancy and birth, contraception and abortion.

- To provide instruction in defining personal values and on marriage, drugs, alcohol, and sex.

- To increase decision-making and communication skills.

Regardless of the specific goals, such instruction is becoming more common, not only in schools, but in churches, youth-serving agencies, and general counseling and mental health programs.

The decision to become sexually active is one of the most important decisions an adolescent will make because of its obvious long-term consequence: parenthood. Yet teens have few resources and few people aiding them with this decision. Many adolescents drift into sexual activity without making a conscious decision. A growing concern about teenage sexual activity, pregnancy, abortion, and childbearing, as well as the emergence of AIDS, has led to an increased emphasis on sex education in the last few years, with broad support for such programs growing steadily.

According to a 1988 Louis Harris opinion poll, 89 percent of adults favor teaching sex education in public schools (Louis Harris and Associates, 1988). A 1982 survey of large city school districts found that 80 percent offered some level of sex education but this was often integrated into other curriculum subjects rather than being a separate course (Sonenstein and Pittman, 1984). Such instructional programs are usually short in duration with most lasting for fewer than 20 hours (Orr, 1982). A 1988 survey conducted by the Alan Guttmacher Institute (AGI) revealed that 80 percent of all states require or encourage the teaching of sex education in the public schools, and nearly 90 percent of large school districts support such instruction (Kenney, Guardado and Brown, 1989).

Roughly 60 percent of teens receive some level of family life/sex education, but only 35 percent of these receive comprehensive instruction in courses that cover at least four of the following six topics: biological facts about reproduction; coping with sexual development; information about birth control; facts about abortion; preventing sexual abuse; and where to obtain contraceptives (Sonenstein and Pittman, 1984).

The AGI survey indicated that public junior and senior high school nurses and teachers of biology, health education, home economics, and physical education believe that a wide range of topics related to pregnancy prevention, AIDS, and other sexually transmitted diseases should be taught in the public schools and should be covered by grades seven and eight at the latest. However, in reality, sex education tends not to occur until ninth or tenth grade (Forrest and Silverman, 1989).

Although most teachers in the AGI survey said that instruction should cover all aspects of sexuality, only eight out of ten of them work in schools that provide instruction in sexual decision-making, abstinence, and birth control methods. Further, while 97 percent of the teachers said that sex education instruction should provide information on where students can obtain contraceptive services, only 48 percent of the respondents said this was standard practice in their school (Forrest and Silverman, 1989).

Much needs to happen to ensure that adolescents have early and ample opportunities to learn and discuss their sexuality and to understand its consequences. Approaches to providing this information include:

- Traditional instruction in family life and sexuality education.

- Social skills-based curricula that help people say "no."

- Curricula that incorporate sex education into a life planning framework or that focus on life skills.

- Training and instruction programs designed to enhance parent and child communication or increase parents' comfort in talking with their youngsters.

- Individual and small group counseling on sexuality.

Programs and Curricula

There is no single solution to the problem of unintended adolescent pregnancy. Many examples of innovative approaches exist in the field, although many of them need to be more fully documented and evaluated, and the successful ones replicated. The programs described in the following pages are meant as examples of a variety of approaches rather than as a definitive set of program models. These programs vary widely along a number of measures, including their sponsorship or base of operation, the length of time they have been in operation, their target group, the ages they serve, the kinds and range of services they provide, and their primary focus. For complete descriptions of these programs and information on their evaluation, please contact the individual(s) listed in the chart at the end of this chapter.

Family Life/ Sex Education Curricula

Whether offered in schools, in religious settings, or through community groups, family life instruction is an important contributor to healthy child/adolescent development. New Jersey, the first state to mandate sex education in the schools and one of the few to have worked actively to implement its mandate, broadly defines family life education as "...instruction to develop an understanding of the physical, mental, emotional, social, economic, and psychological and cultural foundations of human development, sexuality, and reproduction at various stages of growth; the opportunity for pupils to acquire knowledge which will support the development of responsible personal behavior, strengthen their own family life now, and aid in establishing a strong family life for themselves in the future, thereby contributing to the enrichment of the community" (Wilson, 1985). The Lutheran church, one of the religious organizations most involved in providing family life/sexuality instruction to its parishioners, refers to it as "human sexuality education," and defines it as "...learning to live with the expression of one's sexuality in different stages (preschool, elementary school, adolescent, early adulthood, middle adulthood, and later adulthood) and in different dimensions (biological, psychological, social/cultural, and spiritual)" (Task Force on Human Sexuality Education, 1986). Community-based family life education programs integrate sexual learning into the many diverse formal and informal groups that exist within a community. A family life education program in a community setting may cover issues and concerns that range from a parent's apprehension over a daughter wearing make-up to issues of marriage and divorce. Many groups design their own curricula and make them available to various institutions. Several are available for review and purchase including the following:

- The Minnesota-based Search Institute's Life and Family National Demonstration Project is conducting an evaluation of a field test in public schools of *Human Sexuality: Values and Choices,* a curriculum developed in collaboration with the St. Paul Maternal and Infant Care Project. The curriculum designed for middle school students provides 15 units for students and three parallel sessions for parents. In addition to promoting sexual abstinence, the program emphasizes a range of values, such as equality, respect, and responsibility. It has been introduced in about 400 communities in 40 states. Results from the initial evaluation found changes in attitudes and intentions, which were, however, not sustained in a four month follow up. This finding has led to development of a "booster" curriculum to reinforce the original gains.

- *Reaching Adolescents* is a ten-part educational program designed by the American Red Cross to help ten- to twelve-year-olds make the transition into adolescence more easily, while avoiding common pitfalls. The curriculum covers such subjects as self-esteem, values, positive and negative influences, gender roles, puberty, peer relationships, and community resources. The curriculum consists of a leader's manual, unit outlines, and audiovisuals.

One aspect of family life education consists of specific instruction on and discussion of sexuality-related issues – puberty, pregnancy and childbearing, dating, peer pressure, relationships, contraceptive methods and services, rape, incest, abortion, masturbation, homosexuality, etc. The controversial nature of certain topics, however, sometimes means that the discussions come too little, too late. A 1982 survey of large city school districts revealed that only 37 percent provide students an opportunity before the ninth grade to discuss changes at puberty; the percentages are even smaller for sexual decision-making (19 percent) and contraceptive information (11 percent) (Sonenstein and Pittman, 1984).

Several curricula are designed to offer youths an opportunity to explore sexuality issues in depth. A number of these are available to interested groups, including the two examples listed here. Many other curricula and training packages that can serve as components of a broad family life program are also on the market. Some of these are specifically aimed at developing decision-making skills, including decisions about sexuality. The General Resource Directory on page 261 provides you with specific suggestions where you can purchase available curriculum materials.

- *Positive Images,* a training manual for adults to use with adolescents, deals with attitudes, communication, and decision-making, both in general and specifically with regard to birth control. The curriculum seeks to create a positive image of contraception and a positive image of young people who use contraceptives to prevent pregnancy, so that young people will feel more encouraged and capable of sexual responsibility.

- *Adolescent Sexuality: Guides for Professional Involvement* was developed by the American College of Obstetricians and Gynecologists for health professionals. It contains basic lessons, audiovisuals, and handout materials for presentation to teenagers, parents, and community groups on sexual development, sexually transmitted diseases, AIDS, teen pregnancy, childbearing, and adolescent repro- ductive health care.

Abstinence Curricula

During the past few years, many curricula and programs have evolved that are partially based on the traditional goal of sex education – teaching restraint. The "just say no" concept has long been used to help young people who are at risk for substance abuse to develop social resistance or refusal skills. Today, that concept is being used to combat a variety of adolescent risk-taking behaviors, including early sexual activity. This approach is generally most appropriate for younger adolescents – those under 15 or 16 years of age who are not sexually active.

- The *Postponing Sexual Involvement* program, designed by Emory University/Grady Memorial Hospital in Atlanta, Georgia, is an education series created to help young people identify and develop skills to resist pressure to become sexually active. This is not a complete family life/sex education program, as it is designed to do only one thing – teach youngsters to avoid early sexual activity. In addition to covering human sexuality, the program offers sessions on social pressure, peer pressure, problem solving, and using new skills. Evaluation of the program indicates that among economically disadvantaged eighth grade girls, those who participated in the program were nearly three times less likely to become sexually involved by the end of the school year than girls who had not had the course.

• The Boys Clubs of America's *Smart Moves* program helps boys say "no" to alcohol, drugs, and early sexual activity. Using a ten-session model, the program teaches age-appropriate skills. Its four components include "Start Smart," geared for 10- to 12-year olds, "Stay Smart," geared for 13- to 15-year olds, "Keep Smart," a module for parents, and "Be Smart," geared for club staff persons. Smart Moves began in October 1985 with ten demonstration sites, and is now being implemented in more than 200 Boys Clubs throughout the country.

Life Planning and Life Skills

This approach to capacity-building combines career exploration and vocational guidance with decision-making concerning issues of social, family, and school behavior. By helping teens develop, plan, and attain their occupational and educational goals, these programs also indirectly teach teens the value of delaying parenthood until progress toward meeting these goals is well underway. *Whether the programs are implemented in schools, churches, or community groups, the people who use the programs to help teens make decisions about their future are also in a natural position to help them gather information and make decisions about childbearing.* Life skills programs provide young people with strong decision-making and assertiveness skills related to problem solving around sexual behavior and other issues.

• The Center for Population Options' *Life Planning Education* curriculum integrates sexuality education with vocational education. Teens are encouraged to examine attitudes toward sexual behavior, parenthood and future plans, and to develop decision-making and goal-setting skills. Evaluation of the program shows increased knowledge about sexuality, expanded perception of the number of occupational options open to women, and increased awareness of personal goals that should be met before becoming a parent.

• *Life Skills and Opportunities* is a Public/Private Ventures curriculum used in its Summer Training and Education Program (STEP). The curriculum focuses on preparing young people for employment and helping them avoid unintended pregnancy. Unlike programs that address the dual issues of teenage pregnancy and employment preparation, this curriculum is a primary prevention program which attempts to make teenagers employable so they will avoid early parenthood. Research indicates that the Life Skills and Opportunities curriculum has a positive impact on participants' sexual knowledge, attitudes, and behavior.

• *Always on Saturday* is a Hartford, Connecticut program designed for 9- to 13-year-old boys. It encourages abstinence and helps participants cope with feelings, in addition to developing problem-solving and decision-making skills through life experiences. The program provides sessions on decision making, goal setting and problem solving, and addresses feelings about community, peers, life experiences, gender roles, self-worth, and sexual involvement.

Improving Parent/Child Communication

The premise of parent/child communication curricula is that improved relations will prevent and reduce early adolescent sexual activity. Most of these curricula focus on younger adolescents and their parents, and offer a variety of parents-only, children-only, parent-child combination sessions.

- *The Family Guidance Center,* part of the Community Mental Health Center in St. Joseph, Missouri, offers sexuality education sessions designed for parents and for parents and children together. The program's primary goal is to encourage parents to discuss sexuality with their children in a relaxed, enjoyable, and instructive course setting. The center offers age-appropriate sessions for mother/daughter and father/son combinations. The parent sexuality education component is co-sponsored by community agencies, such as the PTA, Girl Scouts, YMCA, YWCA, continuing education programs, and local churches; the parent/child communication sessions are part of a broader sexuality education program for junior and senior high schools. The Family Guidance Center serves nine counties in a predominantly rural area that, since 1980, has seen a 30 percent reduction in teenage pregnancies.

- *Families Talk About Sexuality* is a prevention curriculum developed for use with elementary and middle school counselors. The curriculum consists of four sessions to assist parents and their 10- to 13-year-old children to discuss human sexuality, family values, and teen sexual behavior. The first session is limited to parents only; the remaining sessions are for parents and children together. The curriculum covers puberty, adolescent issues, decision making, and communication.

Individual and Small-group Counseling

In addition to access to sexuality-specific information and services, young people need to engage in a personal, interactive process of discussion with adults and peers through which they can sharpen their values and assess others' values and behaviors. This type of interaction is more easily achieved and reinforced in small, informal groups, and can be found in programs that include such techniques as drop-in counseling, peer counseling, teen theater, and hotlines. Many community-based organizations and family counseling agencies offer such opportunities to teens and parents, either under their own auspices or linked to schools, churches, and other organizations.

- Inwood House, a New York City community agency serving young single women and their children, sponsors *Teen Choice,* a pregnancy prevention program linked with the NYC public school system. *Teen Choice* operates in two junior and five senior high schools in Brooklyn and Manhattan and offers information, counseling, and referrals on human sexuality, family planning, pregnancy, and parenting to teenage girls and boys through semester-long discussion groups and classroom presentations. The program's social workers are available for individual counseling and may be consulted for sexuality- and pregnancy-related concerns, as well as for general mental health evaluation and counseling, family problems, and general social service referrals.

- *Call Fran, Call Gwen* are local (Nashville) and state (Tennessee) pregnancy prevention hotlines for teens, providing sexuality and pregnancy information, telephone counseling, and referrals to appropriate services. Teen callers are encouraged to maintain contact with the hotline, calling again after they have used the recommended services (for example, after they have received results from their pregnancy tests). The hotline staff also strongly advocate prenatal care for pregnant teens who call, and family planning services for all sexually active teens who contact them. The statewide and local lines each average 40 to 60 calls each per month.

- Based on the assumption that young males may be more comfortable discussing matters of sexuality among themselves and, possibly, more willing to heed the advice of their peers, some programs have integrated peer counseling into their approaches. The *Male Involvement Program* is a peer counseling program targeting males ages 9 to 19 in a three-county catchment area surrounding Detroit. Fifteen and 16-year-old boys are recruited from local high schools and community agencies to serve as counselors for boys 9 to 14. The peer counselors participate in an intense 98-hour training course before the school year begins, and then conduct human sexuality sessions for boys in the target age groups throughout the year. Funds supplied by the Michigan Department of Social Services are used to pay the peer counselors $4.25 per hour for time spent in the training sessions and in conducting the workshops.

System-wide Programs

Whatever approach is chosen, there is a big difference between implementing a single program and implementing a program system-wide. The keys to successful implementation or expansion of family life education in systems such as schools are easy to identify but sometimes difficult to achieve: community support, parental involvement, and teacher training.

- The *Family Life Curriculum,* in Alexandria, Virginia, has been successful because of its ability to generate parental approval and involvement and community support, and to provide quality teacher training. The program started in 1980, when a group of concerned parents approached the Alexandria City School System asking for a comprehensive family life curriculum for grades kindergarten through twelve. Working with the parents and the community, the school board designed and initiated the curriculum in 1981. Over the last seven years, the program has been implemented in stages, introducing two grade levels of the curriculum each school year since 1981. The school system also provides and pays for graduate-level courses through the University of Virginia. The training program meets weekly for two and one-half years and is open to all teachers. Although formal training ended with the final implementation phase of the program, teachers are offered workshops and training throughout the year.

Contraceptive Counseling and Services

While early and adequate sex education is vital, it is only effective in helping prevent teenage pregnancy if teens obtain the contraceptive counseling and services they need. However controversial, the provision of contraceptive information, counseling, and services for young people who are sexually active is the key to reducing early, unintended pregnancy. *While a mechanism exists to distribute federal family planning funds throughout the country, the lack of sufficient funding and low administrative priority for the program results in only a small proportion of eligible women, particularly adolescents, receiving services.*

Historically, the Family Planning Services and Population Research Act (Title X) of 1970 created for the first time a national family planning program for low-income women. Because teens' income is considered, rather than that of their parents, basically all teenagers are eligible. Title X project grants are allocated to a wide variety of agencies to subsidize family planning services.

Outreach and counseling are critical components of contraceptive services. Family planning clinics have had a difficult time enrolling and keeping teenage patients. In 1981, family planning clinics were used by nearly five million women, only 1.5 million of whom were teenage girls seeking medically prescribed contraception. In many clinics, only about half of the teenage clinic patients make a return visit (Forrest, 1980).

Family planning clinics encounter problems with enrolling young men in clinic programs and providing them with physical exams and contraceptive services. These clinics are female-oriented, with males representing fewer than one-half of one percent of their patients. In 1978, male involvement was designated as a special initiative of family planning programs, and in 1979, a five-year expansion in services to males was called for and funded with approximately $600,000. By 1980, this special initiative had all but disappeared. The fact that none of those first generation Title X programs for males exist today attests to the difficulty of continuing a male involvement program past the initial demonstration phase. In 1984, a new initiative was launched that allotted $50,000 for each of ten federal regions to provide family planning services to males. The $50,000 was divided among a number of family planning agencies, so that grants for each effort were quite small (Adams-Taylor, Novick, Pittman, and Adams, 1988).

The ongoing concern to involve males in teenage pregnancy prevention is being driven, in large part, by the feeling that if they will not be voluntarily responsible for the consequences of their sexual activity, they must then be forced to take more responsibility for pregnancy prevention. Sex educators and family planning providers have realized that just opening their doors to young males is not enough; many are now packaging information and services around sexuality in ways that are appealing to young men. Some are not just expecting males to come in for information, but are disseminating information and services to them.

- *Three For Free* is a condom distribution program funded and administered by the Maryland State Health Department's Division of Family Planning, in cooperation with the State AIDS Administration. In existence since 1983, the program has nearly 250 distribution sites statewide, and distributed more than one million condoms in 1988. The condoms are distributed by 90 agencies, including community job training, health and recreation centers. One unique feature is that condoms are distributed with no questions asked. This eliminates the fear and embarrassment often cited by young people as a barrier to condom purchase.

Linking Capacity-building Information with Contraceptive Services

Programs that link knowledge-based sex education programs with direct clinic services appear to have a positive impact on behavior. This linkage can occur when information and counseling programs develop linkages to a clinic service as in the Adolescent Clinic and the Health Bridge (see below). It can also occur when clinic programs develop information and counseling programs and more aggressive outreach techniques as in the Young Men's Clinic, Smart Start, and the Dollar-A-Day program.

- The *Adolescent Clinic* in Baltimore demonstrated a 25 percent reduction in teenage pregnancy through the combined use of sexuality education and small-group counseling in the schools, with family planning offered at a nearby clinic site. The program also demonstrated that among teens with three years of exposure to the clinic, the average onset of sexual activity was delayed seven months.

- The *Health Bridge,* one component of the Girls Clubs of America teen pregnancy prevention program, adapts the school-based comprehensive clinic model to include intensive sexuality education. In Dallas, for example, weekly classes are offered by a nurse practitioner on topics ranging from aerobic activity to reproductive physiology. The club has a cooperative agreement with the West Dallas Children and Youth Clinics, whereby girls can visit the clinics to obtain any health care they need, including contraceptives.

- The *Young Men's Clinic,* an offshoot of the Young Adult Clinic at Columbia University in New York City, has been providing reproductive health services to adolescent males since 1985. The clinic works closely with neighborhood youth groups and schools, and includes community education and outreach as an integral part of its services. One outreach technique involves videotaping young men playing basketball on local playgrounds and then inviting them to the clinic to see themselves on videotape. At the same time, they can talk to counselors, receive physical examinations, learn about health and sexuality, and receive condoms if necessary. The clinic attributes its success in motivating young men to use its services, in part, to its multi-service mindset, which the clinic defines as "... being accessible to the young men on a multitude of levels." For example, if a young man needs a physical examination for work or sports, the clinic provides that service, and integrates reproductive health information into the visit as well.

- *Smart Start* is a new program of the Family Planning Council of Southeastern Pennsylvania. It has changed the basic system of providing family planning services to teenagers in a way that increases their access to clinics and improves their ability to effectively use birth control. The program benefits two sets of teens: those who are in need of family planning services because they are sexually active (or are planning to become so) and are unaware of family planning clinics or reluctant to use them, and those who have attended family planning clinics, but do not use contraceptives effectively, or do not return to the clinic for scheduled visits. Smart Start services are provided through six subcontracting agencies. All six have implemented changes aimed at the first group of teens, including: expanding the amount of time spent on counseling and support services, individualizing those counseling and education services to meet each teen's unique needs, and following up on teens through scheduled telephone check-ins. For the second group of teens, four of the six sites will also implement changes in the timing of medical services. Called *Smart Start Plus,* the program allows non-pregnant teens with low health risks to receive a limited supply of birth control pills, condoms, and/or foam (after receiving individual counseling and education at the initial visit) without first having a pelvic examination. The timing of the initial pelvic exam is under the teen's control for the first six months after she receives contraceptives. The intent is to narrow the time delays teens experience in using family planning services, as well as to improve upon the education and counseling they receive about the importance of obtaining medical care.

- *The Dollar-A-Day Teenage Pregnancy Prevention Program* began in 1986 as a program of Planned Parenthood of the Rocky Mountains and the Denver Children's Home. The intent of the program is to prevent repeat pregnancies among high-risk Hispanic teenagers at Mariposa Health Station in Denver. The program identifies young women with at least one pregnancy by age 16 and recruits them to attend weekly meetings at the neighborhood health station. The meetings incorporate decision making and life planning into the contraceptive services the young women already receive. These teens are paid one dollar for each day that they avoid pregnancy. An evaluation showed that of the original Dollar-A-Day group, only 17 percent had a repeat pregnancy by the time they turned 18, compared to a national repeat pregnancy rate of 43 percent in 1987.

Comprehensive Adolescent Health Clinics

Both in and out of schools, comprehensive adolescent health clinics have demonstrated remarkable success in reaching teens and providing services to them. Key factors in their success appear to be:

- Accessible hours and locations;

- Multi-disciplinary staffs trained in delivering services to teens (e.g. nurse practitioners, counselors, health educators, etc.);

- Available services without long waits for appointments;

- Appropriate protocols that take into account socially related health problems, confidentiality, and continuity;

- Integrated health education so that teens know not only what to do, but why;

- Affordable services;

- The provision of an array of services on-site;

- Referrals to other appropriate community providers as necessary.

School-based or school-linked comprehensive adolescent clinics have emerged as a viable, innovative, and responsible approach to effective holistic health care delivery for teens. These school-based clinics (SBCs) have grown from a single site in 1970 to 156 programs in the first half of 1989. SBCs are a small fraction of all adolescent health clinics, but have demonstrated that both young women and young men will use health care services in schools. They make a number of contributions, including:

- Increasing the utilization of health services;

- Diagnosing previously undetected medical conditions;

- Improving mental health;

- Decreasing substance abuse;

- Increasing the number of adolescents who utilize contraceptives;

- Improving pregnancy outcomes for teens who bear children.

Reproductive health care is an essential part of services generally provided by these clinics, but represents fewer than 20 percent of total monthly services provided by

most clinics; the majority of visits, in fact, are related to primary health care or mental
health services. A number of school-based clinic programs provide relatively little in
the area of reproductive health, and the majority of programs do not dispense contraceptives. Nonetheless, even if they do not dispense contraceptives, these clinics
provide sorely needed information and education and are an important link to services
in clinics outside of the schools.

- *The Adolescent Primary Health Care Clinic* provides services to students in eight
  junior and senior high schools in one of Houston's poorest areas. Operating since
  1981, the clinic provides free health care to eligible students and their children. The
  clinic has initiated dropout prevention and service programs that build upon
  medical care and counseling. Housed with the clinic in a converted junior high
  school is a program serving over 200 pregnant and parenting teenage girls, called
  Training and Employment for Adolescent Mothers (TEAM II). TEAM II provides
  child care, medical services, vocational training and placement, and educational
  services to poor young women aged 14 to 22. In addition to the program to aid
  young mothers, the Adolescent Primary Health Care Clinic also initiated the Fifth
  Ward Enrichment Program (see Life Options Programs, page 39), which targets
  young adolescent boys at risk of dropping out of school.

- The Southwest Mississippi *Jackson-Hinds School-based Adolescent Health Program*
  opened at Lanier High School in 1979. Since that time, clinics have opened in four
  additional junior and senior high schools in the rural portion of Hinds County. The
  emphasis is on comprehensive services, ranging from medical and dental services
  to social and psychological counseling. Because of the high incidence of adolescent
  pregnancy in Jackson's high schools, the program counsels students on the
  significant health and socioeconomic hazards associated with teen pregnancy and
  early childbearing. Family planning counseling is provided for those students found
  to be at highest risk for pregnancy, and for those students who are already pregnant, the program arranges for prenatal care through the Jackson-Hinds Health
  Center. In addition, child care is provided for infants of teen mothers to facilitate
  the mother's return to school. As a result of the program, birth rates at Lanier High
  School declined from 65 percent in school year 1979-80 to 16 percent in 1985-86.

Although school-based clinics have received a lot of attention, the model is only one of
many that should be considered in designing a community-wide intervention. Unless
the school clinic has a real commitment to pregnancy prevention, it will not be effective in reducing pregnancy rates. In communities where the school system is not
ready to accept the placement of truly comprehensive clinics in schools, it might be
better to strengthen the family planning clinic delivery system by developing firmer
linkages with schools through formal referral systems, increasing community outreach, and improving the quality of the services provided. Access to comprehensive
health services is only one of the supportive services that high-risk youths need to
maximize the use of available opportunities.

**Enhancing
Life Options:
Creating the
Opportunity
Structure to
Prevent
Teenage
Pregnancy**

For teens with limited life options, teenage pregnancy prevention takes on a broad scope. For these teens to avoid early parenthood, we must simultaneously strengthen their academic skills, broaden their life experiences, improve their health care, provide family supports, and increase their opportunities through education, employment exposure and training, and recreation. In each of these areas, young people need information and support to build their potential for making decisions. For example, they need to find out about the range of available jobs to begin defining their career interests. In addition to information, they need adult monitoring and guidance. In each area of their lives and at each stage of development, young people need appropriate help in assessing their progress, making choices, and identifying and linking up with supports and opportunities.

A range of programs to enhance life options exists. Major strategies that address differences in life options, such as school reform and reorganization, raising the minimum wage, or welfare reform, are beyond the scope of this chapter. Still, there are many other programmatic strategies to improve life options.

*Linking Family Life
Education to Life
Options Programs*

Sexuality education is an important component of the general developmental education that children and youths need, but it is not the only component. Increasingly, sexuality education is included in broader programs that address other developmental areas. Specifically, in several instances, sexuality education is built into school-linked programs that directly address other issues, such as dropout prevention, employment and training, and health concerns.

- *The Teen Outreach Program,* an after-school program of the Association of Junior Leagues, helps teens see themselves as effective, contributing members of their community by placing them as volunteers in community agencies. In addition to the volunteer experience, young men and young women participate in weekly after-school discussions led by a trained facilitator who guides them through a curriculum that focuses on life management skills. Discussion issues include sexuality, self-esteem, career planning, and substance abuse. Teen Outreach is being replicated in more than 50 programs operated by 17 Junior League affiliates and involves more than 1,000 students in the United States and Canada. The program's success is measured by change in five areas: school failure, suspension, dropping out of school, pregnancy, and births. Program evaluation reveals that in 1985-1986, Teen Outreach participants experienced fewer pregnancies, fewer births, and fewer dropouts than students not enrolled in the program.

- *The Summer Training and Education Program (STEP),* sponsored by Public/ Private Ventures of Philadelphia, Pennsylvania, has the goals of: reducing learning loss experienced by disadvantaged students during the summer months; improving reading and math skills; increasing graduation rates; and reducing the incidence of teen parenthood. A five-site national demonstration project since 1985, the program has shown impressive short-term results; data from 1986 show that for the third consecutive summer, STEP participants scored better in math and reading tests than a control group of similar youths with summer jobs only. Participants also revealed substantial improvements in their knowledge of the consequences of various life decisions, including those related to sexual activity. Based on these results, STEP has been institutionalized in four of the five demonstration sites; was replicated in 11 new sites in four states during 1988; and is currently being replicated in 50 sites in ten states at the request of the U.S. Department of Labor.

- *The Fifth Ward Enrichment Program (FWEP)* of the Urban Affairs Corporation (UAC) in Houston is a school-based, holistic approach to health care and education for boys 11 to 15 years of age. Participants are primarily from single-parent households and low-income families, and have behavioral or academic problems. Volunteer tutors work to improve students' math and reading skills; health education and life management skills are also stressed. Boys who participate in FWEP are also eligible to receive services through UAC's other programs; they receive health care, including contraceptives, through the health center, and can receive additional counseling, educational guidance, and employment skills.

Comprehensive Programs to Improve Life Options

There is great support for and merit in developing comprehensive, multi-service programs that bolster teens' life options and motivation to prevent early sexual activity and pregnancy. Examples of comprehensive programs that combine reproductive and general primary health care services with programs in education, employment, and recreation are outlined below.

- *The Dunlevy-Milbank Children's Aid Society Center* sponsors a primary pregnancy prevention program with three New York City sites. The three centers operate simultaneously with program components running in cycles similar to semesters. All facets of the program are offered on two levels – one for adolescents and one for their parents. A family life/sex education program emphasizes taking care of your body. The medical and health program provides physical examinations to all participants and dispenses contraceptives to those who are sexually active. Each participant who is having sexual intercourse is counseled each week by a worker who answers all questions and encourages consistent contraceptive use. The education program offers homework assistance and tutoring after school. Education managers serve as case managers for each student enrolled in the program. Each case manager is responsible for helping a group of students complete high school and, when desired, to prepare for college, since a unique feature of this program is a college admissions component. Every teen and parent who participates in the program who also has a high school diploma or GED is guaranteed admission to Hunter College of the City University of New York. A scholarship fund has been established to supplement financial aid. The center offers several other components, including a job club, an employment preparation class that guarantees jobs to its graduates; an entrepreneurial apprenticeship program, plus a work-learning experience for 12- to 15-year-olds; a performing arts program that enhances problem-solving skills and encourages self expression; and a recreation program involving sports that require youths to master self-discipline and control.

- *El Centro de la Communidad Unida* is a Hispanic youth-serving agency in Milwaukee providing social, recreational, vocational, educational, health, counseling, cultural, and community development services. Through seven program components, El Centro serves a wide range of youths and families. One program at the center, Decisions for Youth, provides bilingual pregnancy prevention and intervention services. Other programs at El Centro include career exploration and employment, a sports and fitness program, a streetwork/delinquency program, a homework center, a cultural arts center, and a drug and alcohol prevention/intervention program. El Centro also offers a training and technical assistance program for other community-based organizations, providing advice on fundraising, research, evaluation, program planning, and development.

- *The Hub – A Center for Change for South Bronx Teens*, began in 1982 as a joint project of Planned Parenthood of New York City and the Bronx-Lebanon Hospital Center. It is a multi-service center that offers 10- to 19-year-olds a range of programs and services designed to prevent too early pregnancy, school dropout, drugs and violence, and to build self-esteem, self-worth and strong academic skills. Components of the program include: the health center, which offers general and reproductive health services, prenatal care, family planning services, and general discussions on sexuality and parenthood; the learning center, which encourages teens to stay in school and offers peer tutoring, computer training, job and college counseling, and a library with information on colleges and job training opportunities; and the recreational center, which offers sports and recreational activities. The Hub also holds community workshops in local churches and neighborhood centers in an effort to involve and communicate with parents.

- *The School Based Youth Services Program,* developed by the New Jersey Department of Human Services, helps adolescents complete their education and obtain skills that lead to employment and additional education, and it supports them in efforts to lead a mentally and physically healthy life. The program's twenty-nine sites are located in or near schools and are managed jointly by schools and other community-based agencies. The New Jersey program serves teens between the ages of 13 and 19 and offers them an array of services ranging from part-time jobs to academic counseling, recreation, and, in some sites, day care for teen parents.

Implications for Program Development and Community-wide Planning

All teens need help in building self-sufficiency, as well as gaining pregnancy prevention information, guidance, and services. Communities should make a commitment to guarantee youths access to the full range of services, activities, and opportunities needed both to prevent pregnancy and to prepare for adulthood. It is also necessary to assist youths and their families in identifying their needs and gaining access to the services designed to meet those needs.

It is unrealistic and perhaps unwise to expect every youth development program that reaches adolescents to take on the delivery of sexuality education, set up small discussion groups, or provide on-site reproductive health counseling or services. But it is realistic to ask that programs recognize that adolescents can express sexuality, and acknowledge and address their needs for sexuality information, even if in informal ways. The same can be said about sexuality-specific programs. It is unrealistic to expect them to be able to incorporate employment training, recreation, or community service activities into their core services. But it is not unrealistic to ask those service providers to be aware that nonsexual issues affect the sexual behavior of their clients.

Both elements – sexuality-specific and youth development – are critical. There is no reason for tension between the two. Community plans should broadly assess needs in both areas; the reality, however, is that if the focus of the plan is pregnancy prevention, capacity-building issues must be addressed. *Adolescents must have access to information and contraceptive services which will enable them to act in a sexually responsible manner.* Because capacity-building issues are controversial, it is easy – especially while trying to build community consensus on action steps – to let these components weaken to the point that the plan can no longer be effective in pregnancy prevention.

Capacity-building issues can be addressed in a variety of ways: through single-focus approaches, such as family planning clinics; within the context of addressing other needs, as in comprehensive programs; or in tandem with other needs, as in programs with an employment and training focus that add on a sexuality-specific component. The extent to which youth development (opportunity structure) is made the focus should be determined by: the extent to which work is needed in these areas; the extent to which your group has the ability, the political will, the authority, and the clout to follow through on recommendations; and the extent to which other agencies or coalitions are already working in these areas.

The community approach should reflect a fit or match among the community's needs, the available strategies, the readiness of the community, and whether or not the community is already galvanized around a particular problem. Some communities may decide to use only one approach, while others may need every strategy available to them. Most communities will need to establish a series of priorities and a long-range plan that determines how these efforts can be phased in, built upon, and strengthened over the years.

Teen pregnancy is a complex issue and not easily amenable to short-term solutions. Many people and resources must be involved for success to be achieved: for instance, a coalition can outline the big picture, detail manageable pieces of the teen pregnancy puzzle, and encourage others to undertake management of specific pieces. Regardless of the approach taken, it is important to be flexible, to do what the community can do well, and keep in mind all the pieces – opportunity structure and capacity – while developing a community teenage pregnancy prevention plan.

Summary

Most people who work with teenagers have long been in agreement that it is imperative for young people to understand the risks and consequences of sexual activity. However, in recent years it has become apparent that many of those who choose to bear children at a young age do so not just from a lack of awareness, but also because they see few alternatives to this path in their lives. Often they lack the motivation or have few opportunities to improve their circumstances. This chapter has concentrated on techniques being tried today to assist adolescents in building the capacity to prevent teenage pregnancy and in gaining the opportunity structure to consider other paths to adulthood. The programs described here provide examples, and can serve as models for new programs. Those who are in the beginning stages of designing and planning community programs are urged to contact representatives of the programs listed here to obtain further information and guidance in their efforts. We urge you to build upon this wealth of collective experience as you begin to consider the types of models that may best fit your community. You may also discover that "hybrid" models may also help to generate the next wave of effort in this very vital area.

Appendix 2-1

Model Adolescent Pregnancy Prevention Programs

Program Name	Sponsor	Contact	Year Initiated	Target	Primary Focus	Service Orientation
Adolescent Clinic	hospital school-linked	Dr. Alan Joffe, Director Adolescent Clinic Johns Hopkins Hospital 600 N. Wolf St., 3rd Fl. Baltimore, MD 21231 (301) 955-2865	1982-1987 as The Self Center 1988	coed 10-15	sexuality educ. & contraceptive services	information, family planning services
Adolescent Primary Health Care Clinic	community organization/ school-linked	Donna J. Bryant Executive Director Urban Affairs Corp. 2815 Reid Houston, TX 77026 (713) 222-8788	1981	coed 10-18	adolescent health	comprehensive
Adolescent Sexuality Guide	national organization	Jan Chapin Assoc. Dir. of Programs American College of Obstetrics & Gynecology 409 - 12th St., SW Washington, DC 20024 (202) 863-2579	1989	coed 13-19	sexuality educ., information & counseling	human sexuality
Always on Saturday	community organization	Amos Smith, Coordinator Hartford Action Plan on Infant Health 3 Arbor Street Hartford, CT 06106 (302) 236-4872	1985	males 9-13	sexuality educ., information & counseling	life skills/ decision-making
Call Fran/Call Gwen	state/local government	Gina Miller, Program Dir. 28 Middleton Street Nashville, TN 37210 (615) 255-2722	1983	sexually active teens	sexuality educ., information & counseling	hotline, counseling & referral
Dollar-a-Day	local affiliate	Suzanne Satter Director of Education Planned Parenthood of the Rocky Mountains 921 E. 14th Avenue Denver, CO 80218 (303) 832-5069	1986	females with a history of at least one pregnancy	sexuality educ., & contraceptive services	information, family planning
Dunlevy-Milbank Children's Aid Society	community organization	Michael Carrera, Director 1432 W.118th Street New York, NY 10026 (212) 369-1223	1985	coed 12-20	life options	comprehensive

Program Name	Sponsor	Contact	Year Initiated	Target	Primary Focus	Service Orientation
El Centro de la Communidad Unida	community organization	Mary Galvin United Community Center 1028 S. Ninth Street Milwaukee, WI 53204 (414) 384-3100	1967	Hispanics coed 12-20	life options	comprehensive
Families Talk About Sexuality	national organization	Pam Wilson, Consultant American Association for Counseling & Development 5999 Stevenson Avenue Alexandria, VA 22304 (703) 823-9800	1987	coed 10-13 & parents	sexuality educ., information & counseling	parent/child communication
Family Guidance Center	community organization	Jean G. Brown Assistant Director Family Guidance Center 910 Edmond, Suite 100 St. Joseph, MO 64501 (816) 364-1501	1976	male-female parallel, 9-17, and parents	sexuality educ., information & counseling	parent/child communication
Family Life Curriculum	school	Jean Hunter Alexandria Public Schools 3801 Braddock Road Alexandria, VA 22303 (703) 998-2160	1981	coed K-12	sexuality educ., information & counseling	systemwide family life education
Fifth Ward Enrichment Program	community organization/ school-based	Ernest McMillan, Director Fifth Ward Enrichment Program 1700 Gregg Street Houston, TX 77020 (713) 223-5108	1984	males 11-15	life options	health educ., dropout prevention
The Health Bridge	local affiliate	Pat Lysell Girls Club of Dallas 5415 Maple St., Suite 222 Dallas, TX 75232 (214) 630-5213	1986	females 6-18	sexuality educ., contraceptive services	information, family planning services
The Hub	local affiliate	Sally Kohn Planned Parenthood of NY 349 E. 149th Street Bronx, NY 10451 (212) 292-8000	1982	coed 10-19	life options	comprehensive
Human Sexuality: Values & Choices	national organization	Shelby Andress Search Institute 122 W. Franklin Avenue Minneapolis, MN 55404 (612) 870-9511	1986	coed 10-15	sexuality educ., information & counseling	life planning
Jackson-Hinds School-Based Adolescent Health Program	local organization/ school-based	Maxine Drey Jackson-Hinds Community Health Center P.O. Box 3437 Jackson, MS 39207 (601) 362-5321	1979	coed	adolescent health	comprehensive
Life Planning Education	national organization	Jackie Manley Center for Population Options 1012 - 14th St., NW, Suite 1200 Washington, DC 20005 (202) 347-5700	1985	coed	sexuality educ., information & counseling	life planning
Life Skills & Opportunities	national organization	Natalie Jaffe Public/Private Ventures 299 Market Street Philadelphia, PA 19106 (215) 592-9099	1984	coed	sexuality educ., information & counseling	life planning
Male Involvement Program	local affiliate	James Wasserman Planned Parenthood 1553 Woodward Ave., Suite 1337 Detroit, MI 48226 (313) 963-2870	1982	males 9-19	sexuality educ., information &	peer counseling; counseling
New Jersey School-Based Youth Program	state	Ed Tetelman New Jersey Department of Human Services, CN-700 Trenton, NJ 08625 (609) 292-1617	1988	coed 13-19	life options	comprehensive

Program Name	Sponsor	Contact	Year Initiated	Target	Primary Focus	Service Orientation
Positive Images	local affiliate	Peggy Brick Center for Family Life Education Planned Parenthood 575 Main Street Hackensack, NJ 07601 (201) 489-1265	1986	coed grades 8-11	sexuality educ. information	human sexuality
Postponing Sexual Involvement	university hospital/school	Marion Howard Grady Memorial Hospital P.O. Box 26158 Atlanta, GA 30335 (404) 589-4204	1984	coed 16 & under	sexuality educ. information & counseling	abstinence
Promoting Action for Teen Health	state/community organization	Elizabeth Roeth PATH Project P.O. Box 876 Helena, MT 59601 (406) 449-8611	1987	coed	adolescent health	comprehensive
Reaching Adolescents	national organization	Rick Walter American Red Cross National Headquarters 17th & D, NW Washington, DC 20006 (202) 347-2852	begins 1990	coed 10-12	sexuality educ., information & counseling	family life education
Smart Moves	national organization	Gale Barrett-Kavanagh Boys Clubs of America 771 First Avenue New York, NY 10017 (212) 351-5910	1985	coed and males only 10-15	sexuality, alcohol, drugs	abstinence
Smart Start	local organization	Dorothy Mann Family Planning Council of Southern Pennsylvania 260 S. Broad St., Suite 1900 Philadelphia, PA 19101-3865 (215) 985-2600	1988	17 & under	sexuality educ., & contraceptive services	information, family planning services
Summer Training Education Program	national organization	Michael Sack Public/Private Ventures 399 Market Street Philadelphia, PA 19106 (215) 592-9099	1984	coed 14-15	life options	sexuality, dropout prevention, job training
Teen Choice	community organization/ school-based	Mindy Stern Inwood House 320 E. 82nd Street New York, NY 10028 (212) 861-4400	1978	coed 12-21	sexuality educ., information & counseling	group & individual counseling
Teen Outreach Program	national organization	Nancy Hoggson Assn. of Junior Leagues 825 Third Avenue New York, NY 10022 (212) 355-4380	1978	coed 14-18	life options	sexuality educ., dropout prevention, youth services
Three for Free	state government	Andy Hannon Department of Health and Mental Hygiene P.O. Box 13528 Baltimore, MD 21203 (301) 225-6727	1983	males 12-20	contraceptive services	condom distribution
Young Men's Clinic	university hospital	Bruce Armstrong Center for Population and Family Health Columbia University 60 Haven Avenue New York, NY 10032 (212) 305-6960	1984	males 12-22	sexuality educ., contraceptive services	information, family planning services

Chapter 3

Community-wide Interventions and Resources for Support

W hile an encouraging number of successful single-focus programs exist, only a handful of fully integrated community-wide interventions are in place. Some communities have established most of the program components, but they remain fragmented and uncoordinated so that in some neighborhoods services overlap, and in others they are unavailable. In some communities, few appropriate adolescent service programs of any type are available, particularly in rural areas. The conceptual framework presented in Chapter 1 reflects the need for developing a comprehensive package of services, ranging from sex and family life education and contraceptive care to enhancing life options. Models for each kind of program were described in Chapter 2. Few communities have attained a level of program development in which all appropriate prevention programs are well established and integrated to create a community-wide intervention. Chart 3-1 shows what this model might contain if all the pieces were in place.

Among the communities that have successfully integrated their intervention programs, several approaches have been used. In some instances, the process involved taking existing individual programs and coordinating them into a systematic formal network. In other communities, a number of new programs were launched simultaneously as a comprehensive pregnancy prevention initiative. Some community models center on the issue of adolescent pregnancy prevention, while others focus more broadly on high-risk youths and include pregnancy prevention as a component.

Included in this chapter are examples of local program models, broad-based coalitions and task forces, and state initiatives. The collective experience yields a number of important concepts that will be helpful to review as your community addresses the issue of adolescent pregnancy prevention. First, however, let us consider the question of fundraising.

Chart 3–1

COMMUNITY-WIDE PREGNANCY PREVENTION INITIATIVE

COMMUNITY INTERVENTIONS	DIRECT SERVICES TO TEENS		
	SEX EDUCATION	CONTRACEPTION	LIFE OPTIONS
• Community education • Media • Parent involvement • Advisory committees • Clergy • Fund raising • Referral arrangements • Community hot-lines • Technical assistance • Library/clearinghouse • Training • Monitoring and evaluation • Research • Advocacy	• Sexuality and family life education • Decision making • Life skills	• Contraceptive services • Condom distribution • Contraceptive counseling • Reproductive health care • Client monitoring	• Educational remediation • Individual counseling, mentoring and support • Education and employment, including job placement services • Life planning • Health services including mental health • Recreation and cultural activities • After school/ weekend/summer activities

The Community-Wide Model

Resources

Individual and community-wide interventions rely on many different public and private sources of support. Most federal and state funding is provided to community agencies through categorical grants – money designated for a specific kind of program, such as family planning, substance abuse prevention, or maternal and child health. With the exception of government supported demonstration projects, there are no federal funds for comprehensive services. Foundations are an important source of support for community-wide interventions with broader goals. However, communities that rely on public sources generally must piece together categorical funds (for individual programs) along with other available program funding.

The major sources of support at the state and federal levels are briefly described here, classified according to the three categories of pregnancy prevention: family life and sex education; contraception; and life options.

Funding for Family Life and Sex Education

With the exception of "saying no" programs funded by the Office of Adolescent Pregnancy Prevention Programs, no categorical federal funds are earmarked for sex or family life education. Seventeen states and the District of Columbia have mandated sex education to be part of the school curriculum. A few state offices of family planning fund curriculum development and teacher training in family life education and

may offer technical assistance to local districts. However, with the exception of the
New York, no state makes available special funds for implementation of these curricula at the local level. Local school districts are expected to use their general funds,
which they may get from the state, to purchase curricula and pay for teacher training.

A recent survey documented that states were much more likely to be involved in AIDS
education than sex education (Kenney, Guardado, and Brown, 1989). More than 30
states and the District of Columbia mandate that school districts provide students with
information about AIDS. Federal funds are available for this purpose through grants to
states from the Centers for Disease Control.

Funding for
Pregnancy
Prevention
Programs and
Contraception

The main public funding for pregnancy prevention derives from the Family Planning
Services and Population Research Act of 1970 (Title X) which helps support some
4,500 family planning clinics nationwide. Since 1978, grant recipients have been
required to serve teenagers. Early in the Reagan administration, the Title X program
was moved out of the Public Health Service along with the Office of Adolescent
Pregnancy Prevention Programs (OAPP) and placed under the auspices of the Office
of Population Affairs.

About $138 million was appropriated by Congress in 1988 for Title X and distributed to
county health departments, Planned Parenthood affiliates, community health centers,
hospital outpatient departments, and a few community-based youth centers. Local
agencies generally receive their project grants through the auspices of state health
departments. A few states also have put line items in health budgets for family planning services and community education. About 1.5 million teenagers use subsidized
family planning clinics every year, representing approximately one-third of all clients
served. An unknown amount of Medicaid and Social Services block grant funds are
collected by local family planning clinics and private physicians to subsidize contraceptive care of teenagers. The use of Medicaid by teenagers requires establishment of
eligibility based on the family's income status, and special arrangements are necessary
to insure confidentiality. However, in a number of states, adolescents can qualify for
sensitive services which are paid for by Medicaid and do not require income eligibility.

The Adolescent Health Services and Pregnancy Prevention and Care Act of 1978 was
the first federal legislation to focus solely on the issue of teenage pregnancy (Dryfoos,
1990). It created the Office of Adolescent Pregnancy Prevention Programs in the
Office of Population Affairs, Public Health Service. The goal of primary prevention was
promptly changed by the program to secondary prevention services for young women
who were already pregnant or were first-time mothers. Thus, for a short time the
limited funds were granted only to local "teen mom" programs. By 1981, appropriation
was folded into the Maternal and Child Health block grants (MCH). Next came the
Adolescent Family Life Act (Title XX) in 1981, the Reagan administration's response to
the problem of teenage pregnancy. A limited amount of grant funds ($10 million) was

awarded to OAPP demonstration projects for promoting abstention among non-sexually active teenagers, fostering family-child communication, and promoting adoption among pregnant adolescents. No provisions were included for contraceptive services.

A number of states have initiated task forces for coordinated pregnancy prevention initiatives. In a few states, special funds have been committed to this purpose, but most interest is in programs for teenage mothers and their babies. In 1983, an Illinois Teenage Pregnancy Prevention Initiative was launched by Governor Thompson with the creation of the Parents Too Soon (PTS) program. Funds from several state agencies were combined to support more than 100 diverse community-based health, education, and social services programs targeted at high-risk 10- to 19-year-olds. The major funding agencies were the Departments of Public Health, Public Aid, and Children and Family Services, with coordination provided by the Department of Public Health. The Departments of Education, Commerce and Community Affairs, Alcoholism and Substance Abuse, Mental Health and Developmental Disabilities, Employment Security, and Services for Crippled Children were involved at the state level in planning and coordination. A major PTS grantee is Ounce of Prevention, a statewide nonprofit agency jointly created by the Department of Children and Family Services and a private foundation, Pittway Corporation. This agency has stimulated program development in agencies for teen parents and pregnancy prevention as well as other youth services, and has sponsored several school-based health clinics. The Illinois experience demonstrates that it is possible to pool state funds and use them to develop comprehensive community-based programs focused on adolescent pregnancy prevention.

Many states are involved in the provision of family planning services through the administration of federal family planning funds, with some states administering funds from line items in health budgets through offices of family planning. Advocacy groups at the state level have been organized around several themes: networks of providers of services to pregnant and parenting teenagers; teen pregnancy prevention task forces; and advocacy for continuing access to comprehensive reproductive health services.

Funding for
Life Options

The concept of life options is so broad that almost every federal and state intervention directed to families and children could fall into this grouping. Adolescents are included in programs serving the overall population of children under 18, sometimes extended through the age of 21. In the health arena, the federal health dollar goes either to reimburse health care providers for services to eligible individuals in various entitlement programs, or to provide grants to states or community-based organizations for a variety of health related activities (Ooms and Herendeen, 1989). Within federal programs, however, the extent and type of services paid for or offered to youths depends considerably on the degree to which the states give this population a priority. For the most part, it is not possible to document how many adolescents are served by public programs, nor how much federal and state money is spent on this population. It is not within the scope of this book to describe all of the resources of support. However, several of the most important sources are briefly outlined here.

*Funding for
Health Services*

Medicaid is a federally aided and state-administered program that pays providers for a range of medically related services to low-income adults and children. At least half of each state's Medicaid expenditures are paid for by the federal government under matching formulas. States operate under broad federal guidelines through which they design and administer their Medicaid services. Thus, eligibility requirements, services offered, and methods and level of payments vary considerably from state to state.

The Early Periodic Screening, Diagnosis, and Treatment Program (EPSDT) is a special program within Medicaid aimed at providing preventive care to poor children. It requires states to provide comprehensive medical examinations at periodic intervals, follow-up treatment, and case management for all eligible children up to the age of 21. In general, states have underutilized EPSDT as a method for delivery and financing health services for poor teenagers, with a few exceptions. For example, Maryland uses these funds in Baltimore city high schools to serve low-income youths.

The Maternal and Child Health Services Block Grant (Title V) provides funds to state health agencies for a variety of services to improve the health of mothers and children, including children with special health needs. Many state programs work collaboratively with other agencies and resources. A 1985 survey of fifty state MCH agencies found most states using Title V and other monies to fund adolescent health services within the parameters of these funds. In 1988, around twenty states had designated adolescent health coordinators at the state level in order to promote the development of community-based, comprehensive health programs for youths. Under a 15 percent set aside, the block grant funds a program of Special Projects of Regional and National Significance (SPRANS), including a number of special programs devoted to adolescent health with an emphasis on service delivery to high-risk and low-income youth. The MCH block grants are administered by the Health Resources and Services Administration, which also administers the Community Health Centers and Migrant Health Programs (Ooms and Herendeen, 1989).

*Funding for
Substance Abuse*

Federal grants from the Office of Substance Abuse Prevention for projects directed toward high-risk youths are also available. This special program was established in 1987 under the Alcohol, Drug Abuse, and Mental Health Services (ADMS) block grant to provide a variety of public education and community prevention services for both alcohol and drug abuse. These projects include a clearinghouse, a program for training counselors and health care personnel, a grants program for projects for pregnant and post-partum women and their children, and a High Risk Youth Model Projects Program, which funds community-based programs for preventive education, early intervention, treatment, and rehabilitation services (Ooms and Herendeen,

1989). Additional funding for drug abuse prevention is available through the Anti-Drug Abuse Act of 1988, which provided the ADMS with funding for programs aimed at preventing drug abuse among runaway and homeless youths, for activities targeted to youth gangs, and educational, recreational, and community-based drug abuse prevention activities.

Efforts at the State Level

Several states have developed initiatives directed toward adolescent pregnancy, pregnancy prevention and other high-risk adolescent behavior, typically focused on preventing school dropouts. States such as Illinois, New York, Arizona, Pennsylvania, New Mexico, Maine, Massachusetts, Rhode Island, and Virginia have established coordinated statewide initiatives on adolescent pregnancy and pregnancy prevention that have the active involvement of several state-level agencies, including at a minimum the health, education and social services departments (Brindis & Jeremy, 1989). In these 9 states there appear to be several key ingredients: 1) leadership either centered in the governor's office or in the health department, with clear support from the governor and/or the legislature; 2) a definite commitment of state funds to the effort, often supplemented by money from the Maternal and Child Health Block Grant and the Social Services Block Grant; 3) broad agency and community involvement, often including not only the state agencies responsible for health, education, and social services, but also labor, mental health, and juvenile justice, with community involvement taking the form of advocacy on state advisory boards; 4) local commitment, achieved by delegating responsibility for implementation at the local community; 5) emphasis on comprehensive services for both prevention and supportive intervention; 6) recognition of the importance of good data collection and case management (Kennick, 1985).

Thirteen other states have statewide task forces on adolescent pregnancy, demonstrating clear commitment and leadership within the health or the human services agency, with the anticipation that the responsibility for implementing task force recommendations will be transferred to the governor's office. These task forces are primarily state funded, although federal funds under the Maternal and Child Health Block Grant and the Social Services Black Grant have been utilized.

Several states have also made a strong commitment to supporting the development and implementation of school-based health centers. For example, the state of Oregon has used state funds to plan and implement 18 school-based health centers, while in Connecticut the State Department of Health Services (DOHS) provided strong leadership in supporting school-based health centers. The DOHS provided $254,000 for seven existing school-based clinics and offered six grants to communities for planning new clinics. That money is supplemented by funds from the federal Maternal and Child Health Block Grant Program, bringing the total program up to $472,000.

A new initiative in New Jersey represents the next generation of efforts directed at providing comprehensive and integrated efforts. In that state, the Department of Human Resources created the School-Based Youth Services Program to provide adolescents, especially those with problems, the opportunity to complete their education, acquire employment skills, and lead healthy, productive lives. This statewide initiative centered within one state agency led to the development of 29 multi-component projects, one in each New Jersey county. The concept is "one-stop shopping" — to consolidate existing services needed by high-risk youths "under one roof." Sixteen of these centers are located in schools and 13 are in facilities located conveniently near to schools. The centers are open during and after school, on weekends, and summers. They provide mental health and family counseling, health services, employment services, information and referral for community services, substance abuse counseling, and recreation. Many provide family planning, child care, transportation, and a 24-hour hot line. The actual mix of services was left up to applicant communities, but each project was required to demonstrate collaboration between the schools and one or more community agencies. Community advisory groups were also required. Funds ($6 million) have been placed in the human services budget to fund these centers, which must also demonstrate a 25 percent in-kind contribution. About half the managing agencies are schools. Medical schools and local agencies, including mental health and health departments, a private industrial council, the Urban League, and a community development organization operate the rest.

Community-wide Pregnancy Prevention Initiatives

Every community has its own unique set of conditions. Thus, no two areas will develop the same solutions to the problems associated with early childbearing. However, a number of universal components have been identified that are incorporated in the models presented here, and these key ingredients contribute to success in the broad experience of integrating community interventions. The appropriateness of their applicability varies among communities, so use them as a guide in your own efforts.

Key Ingredients

1. **Commitment of public officials:** Commitment by local officials and community leaders to the goal of preventing early unintended pregnancies among adolescents, as demonstrated by publicly stated support for initiatives and active participation on task forces or commissions.

2. **Commitment of public funds:** Commitment of public funds or services (as new, in-kind, or matching funds) to the establishment and implementation of initiatives.

3. **Media messages to the community:** A consistent message to young people through the media and other community channels that opportunities are available other than early childbearing.

4. **Access to prevention programs:** Availability of programs that enhance the capacity to prevent pregnancies, including sex and family life education, birth control clinics, and condom distribution programs.

5. **Access to pregnancy options programs:** Availability of pregnancy counseling and related abortion, adoption, and maternity services.

6. **Focus on schools:** A special emphasis on school settings, especially middle schools, where at-risk children can be reached before they drop out. The strong relationship between school failure and adolescent pregnancy points to the vital role school can play in adolescent pregnancy reduction. Additionally, schools can act as a locus for pregnancy prevention programs in a variety of ways, providing sex and family life education, decision-making skills, referrals to community agencies, school-based health centers or school-linked community programs, educational enhancement, vocational education, counseling, and numerous support services.

7. **Priority for serving high-risk youth:** Disadvantaged young people, including out-of-school and homeless youth, require a comprehensive package of services – reproductive health services plus educational enhancement, social support, general health services, homeless services, and job preparation and placement.

8. **Broad-based and strong support:** Support from local parents and community leaders, including both religious and business leaders, is essential to the success of pregnancy prevention efforts. This support from an array of community leaders and others should be on the record, and supporters should be available for comment. Otherwise, small, but vocal, minorities can undermine both the momentum and depth of community plans.

9. **Crisis intervention and referral system:** A network of agencies that provide referrals for adolescents can also include a 24-hour hotline.

10. **Service coordination:** Agencies should work together in developing a system of care that decreases service gaps and avoids duplication of services. In many communities, this includes a designated lead agency that coordinates planning and linkages among agencies.

In addition to the ten components listed above, communities may want to identify other priorities, such as involvement of private industry, development of parent support groups, and/or establishment of support groups for young people to facilitate the critical transition from middle to high school.

The following case examples provide information on how the ten criteria have been used by a number of communities to develop community-wide strategies. Although all ten criteria do not fit each program's circumstances, the criteria are listed here as a way of illustrating their importance to the overall success of the program.

Mayor's Office of Adolescent Pregnancy and Parenting Services, New York City

Background: The Office of Adolescent Pregnancy and Parenting Services in New York City (OAPPS) was established in 1984 to address the high rate of teen pregnancy and the need for coordination among many youth-serving city agencies. The Office functioned from 1984-1989; in 1990 the Office was absorbed into a newly created Mayor's Office for Children and Families. The following description explains the activities of the Office during the time that it functioned independently.

The first step toward coordination was to convene the Adolescent Pregnancy Interagency Council (APIC), a council representing all city agencies that provided services to adolescents. The council identified the needed policies and programs and planned an integrated strategy for implementing them. The resulting planning document, *A Coordinated Strategy on the Issues of Adolescent Pregnancy and Parenting in New York City* (1986), includes extensive data about the trend of teenage pregnancy in New York City, accounts of what agencies are doing, and recommendations for further efforts in sex education, health care, and support services.

1. **Commitment of public officials:** The city served as the lead agency of OAPPS. It was staffed by a coordinator. The council has kept the mayor informed of developments in the adolescent pregnancy field and testified on behalf of budgetary requests.

2. **Commitment of public funds:** Among the recommendations, the plan calls for development of community-by-community needs assessments and local coordinated plans. Community Planning For Teens, a program within the city Health Department, Bureau of Maternal Services and Family Planning, administers one and a half year planning grants to community-based organizations to organize at the local level, conduct needs assessments, develop formal teen pregnancy prevention plans, and seek funding for implementation of the plans. An important component of this program is the provision of extensive technical assistance to grantees. Two organizations produced formal plans during the first round of Community Planning for Teens funding; the second round of funding to three organizations is currently underway.

3. **Media messages to the community:** The "Be Smart About Sex" campaign developed six posters placed in subways and buses to promote use of contraception among adolescents. It also included a library and clearinghouse of materials about adolescent pregnancy issues, and staff responded to numerous requests from the media for information.

4. **Access to prevention programs:** The Office published directories describing available services and eligibility requirements in *Teen Pregnancy and Parenting Services: A Guide to New York City Municipal Agencies; New York City Parent Education Programs* (with services listed for teen parents); and the *Guide to Substance Abuse Treatment Resources for Pregnant/Parenting Adolescents.*

5. **Access to pregnancy options programs:** The Office published a monthly newsletter listing current programs, new programs to be aware of, current resources, and other information to more than 4,000 public and private providers.

6. **Focus on schools:** The Office and APIC cooperated with public interest organizations to advocate for the Board of Education to implement a city-wide family living and sex education curriculum. In addition, the Office and APIC advocated for city and state funds to support school-based clinics in New York.

7. **Priority for serving high-risk youth:** All of the agencies represented on the APIC counsel primarily serve high-risk youth and have as their mandate providing programs for high-risk youth. For example, the Department of Employment has a summer youth employment program targeted to adolescent parents.

8. **Broad-based and strong support:** The Office and APIC worked very closely with the New York City Task Force on Teen Pregnancy (a coalition of community-based organizations and others who provide services to youth which was chaired by a representative from the New York City Comptroller's Office) and the Teen Pregnancy Networks. The teen pregnancy networks, funded by the Department of Youth Services and operating in each of the five boroughs of New York City, have over 100 youth-serving agency members who meet monthly to work on local issues, attend lectures, disseminate information and enhance coordination of services. Each member of the network provides referral information to other agency members.

9. **Crisis intervention and referral system:** The media campaign conducted by the Office coordinated their efforts with the Women's Healthline, a telephone hotline operated by the Department of Health. Thousands of phone calls were received by a hot line number advertised on bus and subway posters informing young people about contraception.

10. **Service coordination:** Twenty city agencies have been involved in planning and overseeing council activities, including the Departments of Education, Employment, Juvenile Justice, Health, Human Resources, Human Rights, Youth Services, Mental Health, and Homeless Services. Representatives attend regular meetings, establish communication between the OAPPS and their own commissioners.

Evaluation: The Office contracted with an independent evaluator to examine the coordination efforts that had been established for New York City.

Further information on the pregnancy prevention efforts in New York City should be directed to: Donna A. Lawrence - Director, Mayor's Office - Office for Children and Families, 250 Broadway, Room 1402, New York, NY 10007

Planned Parenthood of East Central Georgia Program, Jasper County, South Carolina

Background: The Jasper County school system, the Jeremiah Milbank Foundation and the Henry J. Kaiser Family Foundation of Menlo Park, California, requested that Planned Parenthood of East Central Georgia undertake a study to determine the feasibility of helping the Jasper County community with the problem of teen pregnancy. With funds from the foundations, an educator/organizer was hired to plan and implement a three-phase program:

> Phase I - A Family Life Education Program K - 12
> Phase II - A Peer-Counselor Program
> Phase III - A Family Life Center

1. **Commitment of public officials:** Planned Parenthood moved forward on this effort only after meeting with county leaders and surveying teenagers and their parents. The pregnancy prevention program was developed in conjunction with the school system in Jasper County.

2. **Commitment of public funds:** The school board provided both in-kind support and money to purchase a trailer for the Family Life Center, which serves as an adolescent health center and as the office for other program components. Although the program began with funding from both the school district and Planned Parenthood, the success of the program has contributed to the school board's decision to fund the total budget.

3. **Media messages to the community:** The project has received news coverage. In addition, general meetings are open to the public.

4. **Access to prevention programs:** Funding is being sought for a self-improvement summer program called Becoming a Better Me, which will target 6-13 year-olds. Currently, adolescent male support groups serving at-risk males have been implemented at two elementary schools.

5. **Access to pregnancy options programs:** When a teen becomes pregnant, she may discuss her pregnancy options with a health department representative (with parental consent), who visits the Family Life Center once a week. If the teen decides to continue with the pregnancy, she may obtain her prenatal care at the Family Life Center. In addition, a special coordinator works to seek out pregnant and parenting teens who have dropped out of school, and encourages them to continue their education, either through reinvolvement in high school or in an outside program. This position is staffed by the school district, with primary coordination by the school nurse.

6. **Focus on schools:** The intervention began with the development of a K-12 health education program, entitled "Health Skills for Life." The model curriculum

focussed on life skills, including health, nutrition, substance abuse, and decision-making. During the second phase of the program, 25 teen peer counselors were trained to work with junior and senior high school students. In 1987, the third phase of the program initiated a Family Life Center, which is housed in a double-wide trailer on the school grounds. Since transportation remains a critical problem for providing health and social services in this rural site, the center provides a centralized location, accessible by school bus, where other community services can provide services to students and their families. Services include health education, referral, counseling, parent groups, job placement, and support services for troubled teens. While the Family Life Center is not authorized to dispense contraceptives, staff assist students with transportation to the health department where they can obtain contraceptives if necessary. Funding is being sought to support a case manager to coordinate, monitor, and follow the progress of teens receiving services at the Family Life Center.

7. **Priority for serving high-risk youth:** Potential high school dropouts are identified for special services, including tutoring, job skills training, and placement. There is also a tutorial/Big Brother/Big Sister program for middle school students. Students who need special assistance are assigned a peer counselor from the high school to provide tutoring and social support.

8. **Broad-based and strong support:** One of the first tasks of the organizer was to assemble an advisory committee composed of parents, teachers, and community agency leaders. The advisory committee made recommendations and approved action on the three phases of the program. All phases were also approved by the Board of Education and the school administration. They also have strong support from the Ministerial Alliance, the Parent Teacher Association, the Jasper County Teen Peer Counselors, the Parents Association, and the County Council.

9. **Crisis intervention and referral system:** None

10. **Service coordination:** The County Departments of Health, Social Services, Youth Services, the Commission on Alcohol and Drug Abuse, Sheriff's Department, and other youth-serving agencies participate in the Family Life Center, providing personnel on-site. This team effort has been very successful and is being studied by the state as a prototype to be used throughout South Carolina.

Evaluation: Preliminary data suggest that pregnancy rates (both births and abortions) have decreased, while in a similar county with no services they have increased. Vital statistics were analyzed to determine if the Family Life Education Program and the Peer Counseling program altered the teen pregnancy rate in Jasper County. A drop of 23% in the total number of pregnancies, a 15% drop in births, and a 32% drop in the number of abortions to teenagers aged 14-17 were documented in the 1986 vital statistics for Jasper County. (Note: these percentages are based on a very small number of pregnancies, births, and abortions.) Hampton County, a nearby county with almost identical demographics was chosen as a control. This county, which had neither a special K-12 curriculum nor a peer counseling program, demonstrated a 12% increase in the total number of teen pregnancies, an increase of 8% in births, and a 3% increase in abortions, in the same year. Ongoing monitoring of vital statistics data is currently underway to assess whether these trends are continuing over time. Jasper county school statistics also show a decrease in the school drop-out rate. In addition, larger numbers of students are continuing their education by attending college. Before the program was instituted, only 25% of students attended college, and since the program began that proportion has increased to 40%.

For more information: Curtis Dixon, Family Life Center, Jasper County School District, Ridgeland, S.C. 29936, (803) 726-7247

IMPACT 88: County-wide Plan for Reducing Teen Pregnancy, Dallas, Texas

Background: In 1984, under the leadership of the mayor's wife, a county-wide Task Force on Adolescent Health and School-Age Pregnancy was formed, which included human service providers, policy makers, community leadership, and representatives from the business and religious sectors of the community. The Community Council of Greater Dallas (the planning and research affiliate of the United Way) approved establishment of the task force and provided in-kind support, including staff for clerical planning and coordination activities, and office space, phones, computers, and meeting space. The task force met for nine months to develop a three-year plan called IMPACT 88. The Community Council adopted the plan in 1985, and with funding from a private foundation (Dallas Southwest Osteopathic Physicians), established an IMPACT 88 administrative office to help the community implement the plan.

1. **Commitment of public officials:** The task force brought together 175 representatives of business, government, media, religious organizations, civic groups, health and social services, public officials, and the teen population, from all racial, ethnic, and socioeconomic groups. Nine subcommittees were formed to study the problem from various viewpoints: 1) adolescent and family organizations compiled a listing of services for adolescents and identified gaps and needs; 2) business representatives addressed issues of economic impact of teen parenthood; developed child care strategies; and developed a plan to meet employment needs; 3) educators increased awareness regarding needs; 4) community service organizations surveyed volunteer groups about services and strategies to match agencies with adolescent needs; 5) media representatives developed a public awareness campaign to combat sexual messages and inform the community about issues related to teen pregnancy; 6) health providers compiled a list of health services for adolescents and identified gaps in service; 7) religious groups focused on ways to reach adolescents and their families through churches and to increase spiritual education relative to adolescent sexuality; 8) political and legislative groups

gathered information on current legislation and made plans to increase awareness among policy makers on issues; 9) funding agencies explored ways to secure funding for implementing the plan.

These volunteer committees spent almost a year drafting a forty-page, comprehensive three-year IMPACT 88 Plan, outlining eight major goals, objectives, and action steps for concerted attention: expanded recreation, accessible health education and care, housing for pregnant and parenting teens, a county-wide media campaign, family and peer support systems, employment opportunities for youth, sex education in all public schools, and childcare for children of school-age parents. A local group of service providers known as the Coalition on Responsible Parenthood and Adolescent Sexuality (CORPAS) published a detailed statistical report, *Adolescent Pregnancy in Dallas County*, to serve as a needs assessment for the task force plan.

The IMPACT 88 Plan was endorsed by 36 local organizations, and a steering committee was formed, pairing members from the original task force with volunteers from the Dallas Commission on Children and Youth, an established advocacy group. Many activities and new programs in the Dallas area have resulted wholly or partly from this comprehensive fact-finding and planning process.

2. **Commitment of public funds:** The Texas Department of Human Services provided funds to develop a media campaign and to pilot a "Teen Advisory Board." The city of Dallas funded five new adolescent pregnancy prevention case workers (now expanded to 9 positions) and established a program to furnish 50 child care vouchers per year for parenting teens. Due in part to IMPACT 88, the local Head Start program won federal funds to open the first school-based day care facility in the city.

3. **Media messages to the community:** In addition to the extensive media coverage generated by the IMPACT 88 project, a county-wide public information and awareness campaign was initiated to inform teens of the new "Teenline" information and referral service and to provide information to the public about adolescent pregnancy and school-age childbearing in Dallas. TV and radio public service announcements were produced, along with billboards, articles, ads, and two videotapes.

4. **Access to prevention programs:** The city of Dallas funds nine case workers to counsel teens in schools, recreation centers, and family planning clinics. These case workers have also developed a peer counseling program and a male sexual responsibility project, and they staff a "Teen Clinic" at a family planning site. The local Planned Parenthood affiliate developed the Teen Age Communication Theater (TACT), which has been solidly booked for performances since its inception.

5. **Access to pregnancy options programs:** Serving Pregnant – Parenting Adolescent Needs (SP-PAN) trains volunteers to deliver prenatal care, life skills, and birth control education to pregnant teens in the clinic setting. Volunteers also visit young mothers in the maternity ward to encourage follow-up care of the baby. Advocacy volunteers are matched one-on-one with parenting teens to help them access medical and social services after delivery and to encourage return to school. Evaluations have shown that SP-PAN clients keep more perinatal appointments, have healthier and higher birthweight babies, keep more well-child visits, and are more likely to return to school than a comparison group of teen mothers. Unfortunately, no decrease in repeat pregnancies was seen.

   Day care programs for children of teen parents include a city-funded voucher system for teens who return to school, obtain vocational training, or pursue a GED. In addition, there are infant care facilities operating in one alternative and two regular high schools. Future plans call for a network of family day homes located near school campuses to supplement school-based care.

6. **Focus on schools:** The Dallas Independent School District expanded its *Human Growth, Development, and Sexuality Program* curriculum to cover middle and elementary school-aged children. In a school program advertised as "How to Blow a $20,000 Scholarship," local experts from Planned Parenthood and other health clinics targeted high school male athletes and discussed how starting a family before they planned could prevent them from completing their education. The program was enthusiastically received by coaches and participants, and requests for repeat programs have been received from all schools.

7. **Priority for serving high-risk youth:** High-risk teens serve on the Teen Advisory Board that advises on needed services. IMPACT 88 successfully raised funding for a program targeting high-risk youth, known initially as "Youth Impact Centers." Through this program, a new youth center called the "Lemmon Avenue Bridge" has been opened to reach inner-city youth. Other centers are in the planning phase.

8. **Broad-based and strong support:** Teens were heavily involved in the planning of IMPACT 88 through the Teen Advisory Board, consisting of teens from different social service agencies, pregnant and parenting teens, and high-risk teens from area youth shelters. Through the efforts of IMPACT 88 volunteers, the business and private philanthropy sectors have contributed over $1 million in new funds for youth programming, with an emphasis on teen pregnancy prevention. The task force has strong links with local PTAs and PTSAs, which were staunch allies in the expansion of the sexuality education program in the schools. In addition, in 1989 the Dallas City Council of PTAs served as co-sponsor with CORPAS of "National Family Sexuality Education Month," an annual public

education event that includes parenting seminars, public service announcements, professional conferences and teen forums.

9. **Crisis intervention and referral system:** The TEENLINE information and referral number directs teens and their families to available community resources. The phone number is advertised throughout the community, including on posters and billboards.

10. **Service coordination:** The concept behind the "Lemmon Avenue Bridge" involves agencies "co-locating" their services – offering programs or sending staff to the center on a regular schedule. At present, 24 agencies have established co-locating agreements with the Bridge, which gives teens both an informal place to spend time and a location to access services and attend programs. Internal mechanisms are being established to coordinate client tracking and cross-referrals, and to better utilize feedback from teens on how programs are doing and what services are most needed. The Bridge will be a place to pilot new programs, evaluate existing services, identify service gaps, and otherwise include young people in decisions relative to youth-serving programs. As a final legacy of IMPACT 88, the local YMCA and YWCA organizations have agreed to coordinate public awareness and advocacy efforts regarding teen pregnancy prevention. This effort constitutes the first formal joint project between these two agencies in Dallas.

Evaluation: IMPACT 88 performed three levels of evaluation: internal evaluation (perceptions of volunteers), program outcome and community changes, and impact on teen birth statistics. Near the end of the three-year implementation period (1988), an internal survey of the 100 remaining task force volunteers was conducted. The purpose of this internal evaluation was to identify problems and to determine members' attitudes toward the program and their perceptions of how well the goals of the plan were met. The results were mixed. Some members were very happy with the effort, while others were disappointed with what was left unaccomplished, and with the way the task force itself functioned. Many members had difficulty understanding the role of the task force as a catalyst and facilitator of a community-wide plan, versus the idea of "going out and doing it yourself."

In retrospect, the organizers thought that a smaller committee structure and fewer volunteers might have been more practical. Another suggested change was to reduce the number of people needed to implement the plan from 100 to a more manageable number, like 30 or 40. Keeping 100 people up-to-date on activities proved difficult. Maintaining a stable cadre of youth advisors was also a formidable challenge.

The second level of evaluation involved monitoring changes in the community and the development of new programs or redirection of existing resources. Two publications,

"Adolescent Pregnancy: The Big Picture" and the "IMPACT 88 Progress Report," described implementation of new efforts and changes in local, state, and national policies. These documents were published regularly and distributed throughout the community. The evaluation process also turned up a lack of documentation of the planning and implementation process. This would have allowed for replication and served as a resource for other communities wishing to follow a similar planning process.

The third level of evaluation centered on monitoring trends in live birth statistics. A final report, "Trend Analysis: Live Births to Teenagers, Dallas County, 1985-1988," documents both positive and negative results:

- The live birth rate to 15-19 year olds decreased from 88.9 per 1,000 in 1985 to 83.6 per 1,000 in 1988.

- There were improvements in the proportion of adolescents who received prenatal care. In 1985, 16.1% of adolescents delivered babies without having any prenatal care; by 1988, only 12.4% went without prenatal care. In 1985, 34.7% of adolescent mothers received prenatal care late or did not receive care at all; by 1988 that figure improved to 26.4%.

- The birth rate among Hispanics improved significantly: in 1985, the rate for Hispanics was 90.5 per 1,000; by 1988 that rate had dropped to 76 per 1,000. Anglo teens showed a slight improvement (decreasing from 35.7 to 33.1), while live birth rates increased for black adolescents (85.7 per 1,000 in 1985 to 87.4 per 1,000 in 1988).

- Live birth rates for 12-14 year olds went up slightly, from 4.3 per 1,000 in 1985 to 5.3 per 1,000 in 1988, with the majority of these births occurring in the black population.

- There was also an increase in the incidence of repeat births from 25.9% in 1985 to 28.7% in 1988.

Results indicate an overall greater need to target prevention messages to younger adolescents, develop future efforts that focus specifically on cultural, ethnic, and racial differences, and increase efforts to help teenage mothers avoid subsequent pregnancies during their adolescent years.

For More Information: Jesus Sandoval, Community Council of Greater Dallas, 2121 Main Street, Suite 500, Dallas, TX 75201, (214) 741-5851

Life Options
Coalition,
Milwaukee, WI

Background: In 1984, an ad hoc advisory group was formed to conduct a needs assessment, to help Planned Parenthood Affiliates of Wisconsin develop a plan to address problems of teen pregnancy in the Milwaukee area, and to determine what Planned Parenthood's role should be. The advisory group made three recommendations concerning Planned Parenthood's role: 1) continue providing access to reproductive health care, 2) continue to advocate for increased sexual literacy through school and clinic efforts, and 3) take an increased community leadership role for a more coordinated effort to address the issue of teen pregnancy in Milwaukee. These recommendations were put into the Planned Parenthood Affiliates long range state plan.

Planned Parenthood then invited youth-serving agencies in the city to participate in a coalition to further the goal of reducing the high rates of teen pregnancy in Milwaukee through a coordinated and collaborative effort to provide improved life options for young people. The goals of the coalition were to: 1) advocate for legislation for life options programs, 2) enhance service coordination, and 3) seek government support for coalition efforts. The first activity of the coalition was to develop a proposal for state support. Although they were not awarded the money, the process was helpful for addressing the difficulties of coordinating involvement of a variety of community organizations. For example, there was some initial concern among smaller agencies in the coalition that they would lose their autonomy and be swallowed up by the larger institutions.

When the coalition began there was some concern about how to get people who were in a position to make decisions to attend meetings. It was not realistic to expect that the executive directors of every agency would be able to meet as frequently as was necessary. Yet there would be a very slow response to important decisions if there were no regular members. The decision was made that each agency would select a regular member who could respond to a decision within 72 hours. This arrangement resulted in a relatively quick response time.

The coalition developed a comprehensive community long-range plan for prevention and intervention services related to adolescent pregnancy and life options. The Life Options Coalition does not provide direct services, but serves as a coordinating and advocacy organization. One important role is to initiate advocacy activities centered on state legislation, while providing information and technical assistance to legislative bodies, school boards, funding sources, and family serving agencies.

1. **Commitment of public officials:** While Planned Parenthood played a strong and committed leadership role at the beginning of the coalition, it has from the start intended that responsibility be shared. For example, the chairperson for the coalition changes each year, after individuals from Planned Parenthood served the first two years. The coalition has recently been reorganized into two parts: 1) an executive directors group, and 2) a members group, both of which meet monthly to oversee the multi-service teenage pregnancy prevention centers.

2. **Public commitment of funds:** When state support was not granted to the program group members lobbied the legislature both as a unit and as individuals. The Life Options Coalition was awarded a Planning and Action Grant by the State of Wisconsin Adolescent Pregnancy Prevention and Services Board in 1987. The purpose of the grant was to develop a blueprint for county-wide action to reduce rates of teen pregnancy in the metropolitan area. The coalition also received funding from the Wisconsin Department of Health and Social Services for analysis of research and publication of the report, *Preventing Teen Pregnancy in Milwaukee, Report and Recommendations of the Life Options Coalition,* 1989. The report presented results of a study that analyzed both the need for services based on birthrates of 15- to 19-year-olds in each Milwaukee census tract, and also the location of existing services. This resulted in identification of geographic gaps in services to adolescents. Recommendations for policy direction and programming address the overall community focus, the education system, media, professional/service agencies, legislative and funding sources, and the private sector. A total of nine specific goals were established addressing teen pregnancy and repeat pregnancy rates; access to programs and services; completion of education; media participation; collaborative programming; state funding; legislative support for holistic teen pregnancy reduction efforts; and involvement of the private sector. One of the agencies did receive funds for the Adolescent Health Care Clinic. In addition, funds for a multi-service teen pregnancy prevention center were approved in 1989 by both the legislature and the governor. The funds ($500,000 for two years) will support comprehensive centers that provide educational tutoring, family social services, and comprehensive health care, including family planning and cultural enrichment activities. Thus, the coalition has been effective in lobbying for pregnancy prevention funds for the coalition as a unit and for member agencies.

3. **Media messages to the community:** The coalition produced a video tape aimed at 10-to-15-year-olds and an accompanying user's guide with a grant from American Express. The content focused on the consequences of early childbearing and available alternatives in the Milwaukee community. Teenagers were employed to write and perform in the video.

4. **Access to prevention programs:** One agency received money for an Adolescent Reproductive Health Care Clinic.

5. **Access to pregnancy options programs:** The original charge of the coalition was primary pregnancy prevention. However, as the coalition grew, the number of agencies serving pregnant and parenting teens also increased. They are beginning to work on improving coordination and referral among community agencies, in part through case management.

6. **Focus on schools:** One member agency runs a school-based health clinic and a clinic at a near-school site. In addition, some coalition members serve on the Critical Health Problem Advisory Committee, which works on integrating health services and the public school system. Also, the Ford Foundation funded a program to train middle school teachers in the area of sexuality and pregnancy prevention.

7. **Priority for serving high-risk youth:** The coalition has publicized studies identifying areas with the highest pregnancy rates in the city and the age groups most affected. These studies show Milwaukee to have a high recidivism rate and a high number of births to black teens, the highest of any major city.

8. **Broad-based and strong support:** To operationalize the life options model, it is necessary to involve every possible individual, agency, and institution that assists young people in their development. Members include organizations and local agencies such as the Family Service Agency, City Health Department, Boys and Girls Clubs, several community health centers and hospitals, the public schools, the Commission on Community Relations (since disbanded), and others. The coalition has recently incorporated, with a board of directors made up of the executive directors of the major agencies in the coalition. The general membership also includes groups not represented on the board of directors and subcommittees and working groups, which are usually chaired by an agency director. The coalition operates independently and is funded through membership fees. Agencies pay $100 per year and individual members, $25. However, if organizations cannot pay the fee, they make in-kind donations of meeting space, printing, or mailing services.

9. **Crisis intervention and referral system:** Planned Parenthood has a teen hotline staffed by peer counselors. (There are also two other hotlines not affiliated with the coalition.)

10. **Service coordination:** One result of participating in the coalition has been better communication among agencies. In addition there has been a great deal of cross-training – member organizations working with one another to enhance staff skills.

Evaluation: The effects of the community coalition as a whole have not been evaluated. However, individual programs have been evaluated including a prevention video, community presentations, and monitoring of encounters at the school-based clinic. Evaluation is also being considered a key element of the multi-service center, and the coalition is currently working with the Children's Defense Fund on this part of the project.

Contact Person: Paul Nannis (current President of the Board of Directors), Commissioner of Health, 841 North Broadway, Room 112, Milwaukee, Wisconsin, 53202, (414) 278-3521

Committee on Adolescent Pregnancy and Parenting (CAPP), Minneapolis Public Schools

Background: The Committee on Adolescent Pregnancy and Parenting (CAPP) was formed in December 1982 under the direction of School Social Work Services to assess and address the needs of pregnant adolescents and teenage parents within the Minneapolis Public Schools. Twenty-five people representing regular education, special education, and support services were invited to participate. CAPP meets four times a year. In September, they review the current status of programs, identify additional needs, and assign tasks. In January, progress reports are made. CAPP staff do a great deal of work outside of committee meetings.

1. **Commitment of public officials:** The city of Minneapolis has made a community commitment to address the needs of youth. Mayor Donald M. Fraser called for a twenty-year "Focus on Youth" to assure the healthy development of the city's young people.

2. **Commitment of public funds:** Since 1977, the Minneapolis Health Department has increasingly preferred to spend its allocation of federal Maternal and Child Health Title V funding that is available for adolescent health care on school-based clinics. The county, city, and school district also contribute substantially to the school-based clinic program.

3. **Media messages to the community:** CAPP publishes a newsletter, *CLINICARE*, to keep the community informed of school-based clinic activities.

4. **Access to prevention programs:** The majority of CAPP's prevention efforts are school-based programs.

5. **Access to pregnancy options programs:** While the school-based clinic staff are not authorized to discuss pregnancy options with teens, they do provide them with a sheet listing the range of community resources and services. In addition, while the teen is making a decision regarding the pregnancy, clinic personnel provide support, counseling, and nutrition information. Students are referred to the school nurse or social worker for a discussion of their options and assistance in making a decision.

   The PACE program, Pregnant Adolescent Continuing Education Center, provides alternative schooling for pregnant students not wishing to continue in their regular school. PACE offers parenting classes, prenatal education, career counseling, individual instruction and, in conjunction with the Minneapolis Health Department, prenatal care.

   The MICE program, Mother and Infant Care Education, enables school-age parents to continue their high school education by providing childcare, parenting education, counseling, and support during the school day. Childcare is provided at the school or in nearby neighborhood sites.

6. **Focus on schools:** Minneapolis opened its first school-based clinic in 1977. Today the city maintains a complete system of school-based clinics in the seven high schools. A comprehensive health education curriculum is offered by the school district to elementary and secondary students. Topics include: human development and sexuality, interpersonal relationships, family interaction, family resource management, education about parenthood, ethics, and family and society.

   The Teen Outreach Program, TOP, holds coeducational dropout and pregnancy prevention classes for at-risk students to build self-esteem and offer opportunities for community volunteer services.

7. **Priority for serving high-risk youth:** Outreach to Parents: Training, Instructional Opportunities, Networking and Support (OPTIONS) provides educational and child care services to adolescent parents who have dropped out of school. Services include GED preparation, outreach, parenting education, day care, and vocational counseling. Through an agreement with the University of Minnesota, students who receive their GED are guaranteed college admission and a scholarship. Teen Age Medical Services at Minneapolis Children's Hospital provides prenatal care for girls, particularly those out of school, in a private home-like setting.

8. **Broad-based and strong support:** While older clinics no longer have ongoing advisory meetings, the three newer school-based clinics still have functioning advisory committees. Approximately twenty members meet every other month, including parents, students, members of the political and religious communities, and school personnel, to discuss needs for additional services. In one school the advisory committee expressed the need for increased coordination among the support services for pregnant teens, and easier entry and access to these resources. As a result, a school pregnancy team was established consisting of the school social worker, school nurse, and school-based clinic social worker. A liaison committee brings ideas from the advisory committee to the school for assessment and implementation.

9. **Crisis intervention and referral system:** There are several hotlines for adolescents.

10. **Service coordination:** The CAPP network has strengthened coordination among the school system, health services, and other youth-serving agencies. Other coordinating groups have also formed.

Evaluation: The school-based clinics conduct evaluations. In addition, every three years, the state surveys 6th, 9th, and 12th graders on their health-related knowledge, attitudes, and behaviors. City- and school-specific reports as well as aggregate reports of findings are generated.

For more information: Nancy Banchy, Minneapolis Public Schools, 254 Upton Avenue South, Minneapolis, MN 55405-1998, (612) 627-3087

The New Futures Initiative:
The Annie E. Casey Foundation

Background: The New Futures Initiative is a five year effort between The Annie E. Casey Foundation and five cities: Dayton, Ohio; Lawrence, Massachusetts; Little Rock, Arkansas; Pittsburgh, Pennsylvania; and Savannah, Georgia. The initiative is aimed at developing comprehensive strategies for addressing problems of at-risk youth. The goals of the initiative are to: 1) reduce the incidence of adolescent pregnancy and parenthood; 2) increase school attendance, academic achievement, and graduation rates; and 3) reduce youth unemployment and inactivity. In March 1988, each community was awarded a grant of between $5 million and $12.5 million to participate in the five-year initiative. These funds were matched on a one-to-one basis with local funds, of which 25% had to be new money.

The underlying goal of New Futures is to bring changes within and among institutions that affect the lives of youth. The vehicle for institutional change in New Futures is an oversight board in each city known as the Oversight Collaborative on Youth Authority, which generally includes influential decision makers such as state officials, the superintendent of schools, heads of social service agencies, clergy, and local business leaders, as well as parents, students, and representatives of community-based organizations. Although each city has designed different interventions to meet the needs of its youth, a common element in the cities is the establishment of a case management system, which serves as the glue of the various program elements. Ultimately, each Oversight Collaborative will use data generated by the case management system to affect policy decisions.

The Center for the Study of Social Policy in Washington, D.C. is evaluating New Futures. A management information system is being established in each city to gather and evaluate information measuring changes in the three program goals. A second part of the evaluation examines changes in attitudes, values, and self-image among teens, and expectations of service deliverers. The third part of the evaluation involves developing profiles of students to document changes in their lives as a result of New Futures.

In addition, the cities have access to technical assistance from the New Futures Institute, which is managed by the Center for Human Resources at Brandeis University. The Institute offers ongoing assistance in areas such as community involvement, case management, education, youth employment, teen pregnancy prevention, and others.

For More Information: Tony Cipollone, Annie E. Casey Foundation, 31 Brookside Drive, Greenwich, CT 06830, (203) 661-2773

The New Futures program in Little Rock, Arkansas is outlined below.

1. **Commitment of public officials:** The Collaborative had twenty-one members, including the city manager, first lady, school superintendent, representatives from the governor's office, a school vice-principal, executives from the private sector, local foundations, community agencies, private nonprofit organizations, and some adolescents. The plan was presented to and approved by the city and school boards.

2. **Commitment of public funds:** The Casey Foundation required that each community provide matching funds. In Little Rock these were provided by city and state government, private business, and foundations.

3. **Media messages to the community:** No media efforts were developed in the first year, but some were planned for the future.

4. **Access to prevention programs:** This effort seeks to prevent school dropout and pregnancy through the development of a coordinated case management system that targets at-risk youth.

5. **Access to pregnancy options programs:** Pregnant and parenting teens are currently connected with existing programs in the community, though the project would like to provide services on-site in the future. Teen parents can obtain child care vouchers and assistance in locating child care.

6. **Focus on schools:** In the first year of the program, all 7th graders at two junior high schools and 10th grade students at one senior high school were assigned to case managers. The second year students continued to be followed, as new 7th and 10th graders entered the program. Eventually, all junior and senior high school students will have a case manager who will assist them with obtaining tutoring and link them to health and mental health services, counseling, and drug treatment programs. Case managers are available evenings and weekends. They work out of the schools but also have offices at the main New Futures site. Tutoring services are available in community locations. When the tutoring programs began, sessions were held before and after school. However, this did not prove convenient for the students, and the decision was made to bring tutoring services to where the teens live. Meanwhile, efforts are being made to expand family life education for the schools to a coordinated K-12 curriculum. At the high school there is a comprehensive school health clinic with four full-time staff members. Clinic policy allows for the dispensing of contraceptives.

There is currently a pre-employment course available to 10th grade students, where they discuss life skills, decision making, goal setting, and the basics of resume writing and interviewing. In addition, 100 students were placed in summer jobs, some in state agencies. Project organizers expect to call on private businesses in the future to assist in placing high school graduates.

7. **Priority for serving high-risk youth:** Although each junior and senior high school student will have a case manager, there is a wide range of needs. Thus, different levels of case management involvement is planned.

8. **Broad-based and strong support:** During the six-month planning process the work of committees and sub-committees was overseen by a steering committee. Hundreds of people, including parents, community members, youth service providers and teens were ultimately involved in the process. Also the foundation requirement of matching funds demanded community involvement and support. A community volunteer mentoring program is planned, targeted at 11th graders to provide support and assist students in planning for life after high school graduation.

The case manager program has established a youth council to provide feedback on case management services and bring up additional issues. Case managers select one individual from their caseload of fifty to serve on the council. Their input has proved valuable. For example, one young member of the council recalled a recent conversation with a friend. This friend and her boyfriend had been having sex. When they talked about it they finally realized that neither one wanted to have sex but both thought the other expected it. Because of a need brought to light by the youth council member, a new program will begin this year to assist teen couples in improving relationships and communication skills. This will be run out of the school health clinic and will be staffed by a mental health counselor provided by a community agency.

9. **Crisis intervention and referral system:** New Futures is currently working with a nonprofit agency to establish a hotline to cover all topics. It will be staffed by teens, supervised and backed up by trained adults.

10. **Service coordination:** The case manager's role is to link the student to needed existing services in the community.

Evaluation: The Center for the Study of Social Policy in Washington, D.C. is evaluating New Futures. The program plan is for five years. Additional funding will be sought for program components that appear to make the largest impact.

For more information: Don Crary, New Futures for Little Rock Youth, 209 West Capitol, Little Rock, Arkansas 72201, (501) 374-1011

*The Montana
Coalition of Healthy
Mothers, Healthy
Babies:
Promoting Action
for Teen Health
(PATH) Project*

Background: The Montana Coalition of Healthy Mothers, Healthy Babies (HMHB) was initiated in 1984 with a group of individuals concerned about maternal/child health in Montana. Promoting Action for Teen Health (PATH), one of several coalition projects, focuses on promoting healthy behavior and decreasing high-risk behavior in the adolescent and pre-adolescent years. In 1987, the Henry J. Kaiser Family Foundation provided extensive funding for the PATH project. Additional monies were received in 1988 from the Northwest Area Foundation.

The overall goal of the PATH Project is to decrease the incidence of adolescent health problems, with a special emphasis on teen pregnancy. Healthy Mothers, Healthy Babies believes the goal of the PATH Project is best accomplished through the building of state and local coalitions that: 1) broaden the base of support and influence for all program activities; and 2) provide hope for the survival of effective interventions. Through local coalitions, the PATH Project seeks to reduce adolescent pregnancy by organizational and direct service interventions at both the state and local levels.

Through the PATH Project, HMHB provides technical and financial assistance to local communities whereby they can conduct needs assessments, establish coalitions and develop prevention/intervention projects. There are now seven community coalitions up and running. Each community is encouraged and assisted to identify its own particular needs, skills and resources. In addition to start-up funding provided by HMHB, each community is assisted in seeking other financial and in-kind support for the planning and implementation of the identified project.

1. **Commitment of public officials:** The PATH Interagency Committee is composed of 12 representatives from 7 agencies of state government that serve youth. The mission of the Interagency Committee is to activate state government to enhance the health and well-being of Montana's youth by promoting awareness within state governmental agencies and acting as an advisory committee to them.

    Through the networking efforts of the Interagency Committee, HMHB has been recognized as a powerful advocate for youth. HMHB staff and board members have been invited to serve on the Governor's Welfare Reform Health Subcommittee, the Governor's Access to Care Committee, the Maternal/Child Health Subcommittee of the Deputy Directors Task Force and the Montana Department of Family Services Prevention Roundtable. In addition, the staff has presented information on teen pregnancy prevention to state agency directors, and information on coalition building to the Prevention Subcommittee of the Deputy Directors Task Force.

    The Interagency Committee is developing a state children/youth data compendium to identify the status of Montana children and youth — their unique capabilities as well as their specific needs. This compendium will assist in the informed planning process of Montana's public officials as well as private agencies.

2. **Commitment of public funds:** Although the PATH Project does not directly receive federal or state funds, many collaborative efforts have been supported by state monies. The State of Montana is one of the corporate sponsors for the Baby Your Baby public awareness campaign, aimed at encouraging pregnant women of all ages to seek early and continuous prenatal care. In 1989, HMHB surveyed adolescents in 19 junior and senior high schools throughout the state. Implementation of this survey and dissemination of the results are funded by a collaborative effort by HMHB, the Office of Public Instruction, and the Montana Department of Health and Environmental Sciences. A conference held in the fall of 1989, "Dimensions of Holistic Development: A Native American Perspective," was jointly funded by HMHB and the Montana Department of Family Services.

3. **Media messages to the community:** The PATH project has developed a 3 year communications plan to create action in solving adolescent high risk behavior. The goal for PATH is to provide a visible umbrella for organizations and community coalitions to promote responsible decision making in teen related health issues. The first year objective was to create an awareness of the issues affecting teen health, the second year objective was to create a demand for action, and the third year public relations objective is to provide a visible umbrella for organizations and community coalitions to promote responsible decision making in teen related health issues.

   Projects have included developing various print and electronic media, participating in media programs and events, conducting and publicizing a statewide poll of Montana voters on adolescent health issues, assisting local projects in developing public relations plans, and developing a modular speakers kit.

4. **Access to prevention programs:** The PATH Project has been instrumental in getting information to people in isolated, rural communities regarding the availability of resources. An MCH resource directory was printed in September of 1988. The resource directory includes information on agencies dealing with adolescent parenting, adolescent pregnancy/prevention, family planning, nutrition, sexually transmitted diseases, substance abuse and support groups.

   PATH Task Force volunteers are currently preparing a "Youth Yellow Pages" directory for adolescents, parents and teachers. The directory will give information regarding the types of activities and services available for youth and can be adapted by communities throughout the state. Local community projects present workshops aimed at prevention such as Parents and Adolescents Can Talk (PACT) programs, assertiveness training, decision making, refusal skills, and sexuality information.

5. **Access to pregnancy options programs:** The PATH philosophy statement underscores the obligation of the health/medical community to provide all adolescents appropriate, accessible, affordable, comprehensive and confidential health care. Local communities are encouraged to include family planning and other health professionals in their coalitions.

6. **Focus on schools:** PATH Project volunteers worked with educators to author the new Montana accreditation standards and model learner goals for a K-12 comprehensive health curriculum. The Montana legislature subsequently mandated the adoption of the accreditation standards by local school districts.

   School districts were encouraged to adopt the model learner goals, but it was not mandated. PATH volunteers have been working with their local school boards to encourage adoption of these goals. In addition, most community projects work closely with the local schools. Some projects have developed and implemented school health curricula. Project Choice and the Young Parents' Education Center in Great Falls developed a video featuring an eighth grade class listening to the stories of four teen parents. The video has been marketed statewide for inclusion in other health enhancement curricula.

7. **Priority for serving high-risk youth:** The PATH Project promotes early identification of and intervention with high-risk youth. During the 1988-1989 school year, a comprehensive adolescent health survey was conducted with a representative sampling of 7th, 9th and 12th grade students throughout the state. The survey was funded by the Henry J. Kaiser Family Foundation as part of their ongoing Community Health Promotion Evaluation Program. Funding for the project was also received from the Montana Office of Public Instruction and the AIDS, Perinatal and Family Planning Programs of the Montana Department of Health and Environmental Sciences. The survey provides baseline data for Montana professionals who work with youth.

   Native American youth are considered to be a high-risk group in Montana by virtue of their economic situations and family dynamics. To address the needs of Native American families, the PATH Project receives counsel from an Indian Advisory Group, composed of representatives from Montana's seven Indian reservations, the Montana Indian Health Service and the Montana Office of Indian Affairs. The Indian Advisory Group meets bi-monthly for education, networking and action planning.

   All seven PATH projects identify adolescents with high-risk behaviors and provide individual or group education and counseling. Two of these projects are located on Indian reservations.

8. **Broad-based and strong support:** The PATH Project emphasizes coalition building to assist communities in identifying teen health needs and developing strategies for addressing these needs. On the state level, coalitions are formed with state agencies as well as private organizations. HMHB has served as a model for bringing people together who share a common interest and cooperatively act upon that shared interest.

   Local coalitions are encouraged to include people of diverse philosophies and backgrounds who can agree on a common purpose. The cooperative spirit generated by local coalitions serves as a model for community development.

9. **Crisis intervention and referral system:** HMHB staff provide technical assistance, resource information, and tools for assessing community needs and planning appropriate interventions. In addition, HMHB provides funding for innovative PATH projects on a local level. The Helena Teen Coalition has developed a high-risk assessment tool to use in interviewing teen clients of family planning clinics. High-risk youth are provided with individualized education and counseling. The Great Falls PATH Project, "Project Choice," has developed a Teen Hotline in conjunction with the Community Hotline. The hotline is advertised and promoted in high school newspapers as well as through posters and stickers.

10. **Service coordination:** HMHB realizes that services must be coordinated to avoid duplication and/or fragmentation and to conserve economic and human resources. HMHB facilitates service coordination with other state and private agencies and encourages local community projects to follow suit. HMHB is actively promoting prevention/intervention activities during the early childhood years, since a healthy childhood in itself promotes teen health. In this promotion of early childhood care, education and development, HMHB is coordinating services with the Montana Department of Family Services, the Montana Office of Public Instruction, the Early Childhood Education project of Montana State University, Parents Anonymous, and the Montana Council for the Prevention of Child Abuse.

Evaluation: The HMHB PATH Project has been chosen as one of four projects in the country to receive evaluation assistance from Social Research Applications of Los Altos Hills, California. State aggregate data from the previously mentioned adolescent health survey will serve as baseline data for teen attitudes and behaviors in health-related issues. It is anticipated that the survey will be repeated every other year for 10 years to determine changes in baseline data. PATH's media consultant has also conducted telephone surveys of adults to assess community awareness of and attitudes surrounding teen pregnancy. This type of survey will also be repeated in the future to determine changes and/or trends. In addition, tools have been developed to assist local coalitions with process evaluation.

For More Information:, D. Elizabeth (Bozdog) Roeth, PATH Project, P.O. Box 876, Helena, MT 59624, (406) 449-8611

Summary

This chapter opened with a discussion of ten universal components identified as key ingredients to be included in any comprehensive community-wide intervention. Community groups are urged to use this list as a base from which to develop their own list of basic components. In the same way, it is possible to utilize the information about state and federal funding agencies included in this chapter to determine those sources most suitable to a particular community's circumstances. The seven case examples that followed this discussion have been outlined in terms of how they meet the ten criteria listed as key ingredients. Their funding sources are also discussed because this demonstrates the varied routes that communities may take, depending upon their needs and goals and the funding channels that are available. It also demonstrates how a combination of funding sources can help initiate and support programs on an ongoing basis.

Readers of this manual may select particular programs outlined here that faced challenges similar to those found in their own community and use these examples as models. For each program, contact persons and addresses are listed to assist readers in exploring these models more thoroughly by arranging meetings, gathering additional written materials, and by visiting programs to observe them in action. Information gathering is particularly important at this stage because relatively little evaluation data exist, and because the programs that have been studied demonstrate both positive results as well as some definite limits to their successes. In many cases there has been less than the expected success in meeting program goals because the program intervention itself has not been powerful enough to result in a more dramatic change. In response to such results, many of these programs are just beginning to institute modifications to address problem areas. It is also important to keep in mind your community's expectations of program results as weighed against the strength and level of intervention and the duration of the program you are planning to set up.

How to Develop a Community-wide Adolescent Pregnancy Prevention Initiative

Chapter 4

Getting Started: The Coalition and the Lead Agency

*I*n many communities across the country, individuals and organizations are working toward developing community-wide initiatives for adolescent pregnancy prevention. As we saw in the previous chapter, some communities are well along in the process. This manual can assist these communities to realize their final goals. Other communities are just becoming aware of a need to address the issue of adolescent pregnancy prevention. Those communities can apply the information in this manual to the very early stages of the planning process, and to every step along the way. Users may be single individuals or agencies, or groups of individuals or agencies who have come together because of a common concern about young people in the community. Although some of the underlying issues have broad application, every community is different, and thus the use of this material will vary according to the circumstances of the communities in which it is applied.

Experience has shown that a single agency working alone often has a difficult time bringing together all the players and resources necessary to develop a community-wide strategy. We will present a model of program planning, development, and evaluation for a community-wide strategy. Our model begins with the formation of a coalition of agencies.

A number of steps must be considered:

1. Putting together the coalition

2. Designating a lead agency and a coordinator

3. Conducting a needs assessment

4. Reaching consensus on the package of strategies to be undertaken within the coalition and in the community

5. Developing a community-wide implementation plan and assigning responsibilities for carrying out its specific components

6. Procuring funding for implementing the strategies

7. Monitoring the implementation process

8. Evaluating the impact of the various strategies that have been implemented and tested

This chapter focuses on the first two steps: putting together the coalition, and designating a lead agency and coordinator. Chapter 5 reviews how to conduct a needs assessment. Chapter 6 focuses on developing an implementation plan. Chapter 7 discusses monitoring its implementation and procuring the necessary funding, and Chapter 8 discusses how to conduct an evaluation.

Putting Together a Broad-based Coalition for Pregnancy Prevention

The previous chapters have described the complexity of the problem of teenage pregnancy, and have demonstrated that no one community sector can solve the problem alone. The diverse aspects of the requisite solutions demand that a wide range of agencies be involved: schools, parent groups, health agencies, youth-serving agencies, community service organizations, media, and businesses, all working closely with youths and their parents. The common denominator is concern about the future of young people and a desire to enhance their chances to grow into responsible adults.

Structure of a Community-wide Coalition

Although a number of organizational models can be adopted, we suggest an approach that involves bringing together a large coalition, establishing a smaller body for oversight, such as a board of directors or steering committee, and appointing a lead agency with a coordinator to implement the work of the coalition. (See Chart 4-1.) In some areas, it may be possible for the coalition to incorporate, and directly hire a coordinator. In that case, the coalition is also the lead agency.

It will simplify the planning process if a lead agency can be designated at the outset. This agency must be acceptable to all potential participants, be free of institutional bias, and have strong administrative capacities. One model for a lead agency is the Mayor's Office of Adolescent Pregnancy and Parenting Services in New York City. (See Chapter 3.) It staffs an Interagency Council on Adolescent Pregnancy that brings together representatives of 20 city agencies for planning and interagency communication. Voluntary community organizations and business interests are not represented on the Council but work closely with the office on collaborative projects. Another example of interagency coordination is demonstrated by the Life Options Coalition of

Chart 4-1   # Development of an Organizational Structure

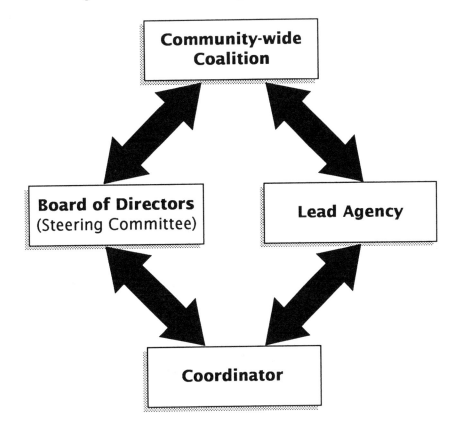

Functions of Each Organizational Component

Community-wide Coalition:
- Sets mission
- Appoints or elects steering committee or board of directors
- Helps design programs
- Helps identify financial and other resources and obtain funding
- Monitors progress on goals and objectives
- Serves as community advocate for action strategies
- Actively participates in the implementation of community strategies

Board of Directors or Steering Committee:
- Helps establish goals and objectives
- Designates lead agency and coordinator
- Oversees work of coordinator
- Designates committees and chairs to work on specific issues

- Oversees work of committees
- Monitors progress on implementing community strategies
- Oversees development of an evaluation plan

Lead Agency :
- Conducts needs assessment and coalition planning activities
- Coordinates work committees and performs the work of the steering committee and of the coalition
- Facilitates functioning of the steering committee
- Helps to implement evaluation process

Coordinator:
- Carries out lead agency functions
- Supervises staff
- Maintains liaison with community agencies

Greater Milwaukee. (See Chapter 3.) This organization is managed by a twelve-member steering committee comprised of top representatives from health, religious, social service, and educational organizations.

An ideal lead agency would have the support of the city government, include representatives from both the public sector (schools, health departments, etc.) and the private sector (community-based voluntary organizations, businesses, etc.) and be in a position to receive and allocate funds from both public and private sources. A mayoralty appointed commission might serve as a good lead agency as long as the *governing board is broadly representative.* An existing nonprofit social agency, such as a community planning organization, Urban League, or United Way could also serve in this capacity. The functions of the organizational components are outlined in Chart 4-1.

The amount of responsibility will vary in each level of leadership. All four levels (coalition, steering committee or board of directors, lead agency, and coordinator) are important, but they represent different levels of community development and consensus regarding adolescent pregnancy prevention. Coalition members will share the decision-making power, usually equally, and share the responsibility for implementation. Members of the board of directors (steering committee) often are given the power to veto decisions, make suggestions, and provide guidance, but they do not do the day-to-day work, nor are they involved in the daily decision making of the coordinator and lead agency. Those communities which have a clear plan of action, as well as the funds to support the efforts, will most likely choose a board of directors. Meanwhile those communities that are just beginning to plan may rely more extensively on a task force or ad hoc steering committee.

Demonstrating Community-wide Support

From your experience in the community, you can probably generate a list of agencies and interest groups that ought to be involved in a community coalition. However, before you start to organize a meeting, there are a number of important points to think about in developing a truly community-wide intervention (see also Appendix 4–1):

• Community "ownership" is a crucial element for program success. Decision makers within the community (both formal and informal leaders) must first agree that there is a teen pregnancy problem. The people whose lives will be affected by intervention efforts will need to "buy into" the statement of the teenage pregnancy problem and the proposed solutions. In many communities today, the sense of alienation and powerlessness is so extensive that even when programs are developed they are not utilized. Community-wide interventions designed with sensitivity can empower potential participants to get involved with the specific issues, and even to work together on broad community problems. In other words, community interventions have to be truly community-based.

• You will need to demonstrate broad community support when seeking funding

Chart 4-2

Examples of Agencies and Individuals to Include in a Broad-based Coalition on Adolescent Pregnancy Prevention

- Representatives from the field of education, including public and private schools, administrators, teachers, boards of education, and university researchers

- Local, county, state, and federal departments (as appropriate) responsible for programs and activities in the areas of health, human resources, social services, child welfare, and public income supports, including Aid to Families with Dependent Children (AFDC), social block grants, and foster care

- Private, community-based agencies providing services for children and their families

- Adolescent health programs and family planning agencies

- Medical societies, including the American Association of Pediatrics and the American Association of Obstetricians and Gynecologists

- Juvenile justice agencies

- Community organizations (PTA, League of Women Voters, American Association of University Women, etc.)

- Community and state colleges and universities

- Major employers

- Chamber of Commerce

- Umbrella-type planning organizations, such as United Way, city or regional planning agencies

- Youth or child advocacy organizations

- Community action agencies, health and welfare councils

- Youth-serving agencies, such as Boys Clubs, Girls Clubs, Boy Scouts, Girl Scouts, Camp Fire, YWCA and YMCA

- Civil rights and minority social service organizations, such as the Urban League, Delta Sigma Theta, League of United Latin American Citizens

- Existing adolescent pregnancy coalitions, networks, or programs operating in your community, county, or state

- Churches, synagogues, and religious organizations such as Catholic Social Services, Salvation Army, Lutheran Social Services, Council of Jewish Women

- Recreational programs

- Libraries

- Women's organizations, such as the Junior League, Zeta Phi Beta Sorority

- Youth representatives

from local, state, and federal school and health funding sources and from private foundations. You will also have to document that community needs are being served, that local values have been considered, and that proposed efforts respond realistically to existing gaps.

- You will need the commitment and financial support of a great many individuals and agencies within the broader community, such as the mayor, the city council, or other decision-makers and leaders. Aim for in-kind support from the health department, school system, community-based agencies, businesses, media, and volunteers.

- There will be certain times when it is particularly important to demonstrate broad support: for example, while conducting the needs assessment; when informing the community about the dimensions of the adolescent pregnancy problem; and when you launch your implementation plan.

- Recognition of the linkage in your community between the prevention of teen pregnancy and the prevention of other youth problems, such as school dropout, lack of employment, and delinquency, will help shape and broaden membership in the coalition. Other task forces may already exist, for example on adolescent health or school reorganization, and consideration must be given as to how a new coalition would relate to these ongoing efforts.

It is extremely important to include a wide range of agencies in your community-wide coalition. Plan to invite policymakers from all agencies serving youth. It is particularly important to ensure non-duplication of services, and comprehensive planning and programing. Chart 4–2 lists the kinds of agencies that have been included in the most successful models. Major categories include the education sector, health care sector, business community, clergy and religious organizations, local government leaders, community leaders, volunteer and civic groups, media, youth-serving agencies, and consumers (including adolescents and their families). Although every community is different, it is vital to the strength of the coalition that the kinds of agencies that are invited to participate reflect every facet of adolescent pregnancy prevention.

It is important to identify other coalitions in your community. As the issue of adolescent pregnancy prevention touches so many areas affecting youth, including education, employment, and juvenile delinquency, you may find that your interests are closely aligned to those of other coalitions. Explore whether initiating a new coalition is necessary, or whether your efforts in the area of adolescent pregnancy prevention could be incorporated in the existing coalitions without diluting your emphasis. If you decide to initiate a new coalition, be sure to establish close working relationships with existing ones. It may also be useful to make contact with other coalitions in your community that do not have a youth focus, such as coalitions working on issues that affect senior citizens. Coalitions may provide each other with support in advocating for their agendas.

Although collaboration among agencies is challenging, both in terms of time and staff resources, there are clear advantages in having community-wide ownership, and joint commitment to actions that emerge as part of the planning process. Collaborative coalitions may also find that the planning process lends itself to a multi-phase action, where specific components may be spearheaded by different agencies.

Given the potentially sensitive nature of establishing adolescent pregnancy prevention approaches, specifically those programs that include access to reproductive health services, some of the strongest opponents to these services may want to participate in the planning process. The lead agency, in conjunction with the coalition, will need to make specific decisions about who will be invited to participate and about the role of each participant. In addition, the governing structure can establish the necessary checks and balances to facilitate group process. For example, in San Jose, California, during the development of school-based health centers, individuals representing groups in support of access to abortion, as well as individuals opposing abortions, were involved in the planning advisory board. While there were many areas of agreement between the two groups, there was much debate regarding what counseling services would be made available to adolescents facing an unintended pregnancy. As a result of numerous discussions and votes on the issue by the fuller community board, referrals for abortion, as well as adoption and prenatal care services, were listed in the clinic brochure.

The Steering Committee or Board of Directors

Once the coalition has been established and a lead agency has been designated, a board, steering committee, or commission can be appointed or elected. Community leaders and important spokespersons for local groups are essential members. The board or steering committee should reflect the community in terms of sex, race/ethnicity, and socioeconomic background. Each community has a different configuration, but in general, members of the following groups can be included on the board of directors:

- Public officials

- School officials

- Public and private health service providers

- Family planning providers

- University researchers

- Youth serving agencies

- Social agencies

- Parents and students, including pre-adolescents

- Media

The board should ideally consist of between six and ten members, and should not exceed fifteen people, otherwise it becomes difficult to plan meetings. All board procedures should be carefully documented and agreed upon by coalition members, as the board works closely with the lead agency in implementing the goals and objectives of the broader coalition. The coalition should also establish whether other members of the coalition may attend board meetings, even if they have no formal voting power.

Members of this steering committee or the board of directors should be:

- Strongly committed to the task and effort

- Willing to provide a substantial time commitment

- Able to assist in reducing logistical barriers

- Able to provide constructive feedback as the program plan is being developed and implemented.

The strength of your community-wide coalition will depend heavily on the effectiveness of the board or steering committee in working with the lead agency and coordinator, and in organizing working committees. In some models, the steering committee operates as an advisory committee to an ongoing effort (such as a mayor's office for prevention of adolescent pregnancy), while in other communities, the steering committee comprises the major work force for planning and implementing the community-wide strategic plan. Steering committee members can help gather information, help the lead agency identify key individuals to interview, select successful program models, find informal community leaders who can enhance community acceptance of the plan, and identify other community resources.

You will most likely find that many service providers and other professionals in your community are interested in the efforts of your coalition. You can involve potential participants in a number of working committees. It is important to keep them well informed of the planning process so that they can feel part of the effort. Hold special informational meetings, for example, with teachers, school administrators, and social service personnel, to address concerns, impart information, and familiarize participants with the special activities of the coalition. As an alternative to public meetings, you may periodically write a brief summary of the coalition's efforts and widely distribute this as a memo or newsletter. If you hold open forums and information sessions you may find that there will be both supporters of your program and those who fear or oppose it. Anticipate any potential controversial issue that may arise and prepare ways to respond to these concerns.

Orchestrating public and private cooperation on social issues is never easy, even when all the players are well-intentioned. Interagency rivalries, turf battles, and narrow definitions of problems all make collaboration difficult. Clearly, coordination and communication are necessary in order to address the complex issues affecting children and youth.

Designating a Lead Agency

It is important to designate a particular group or agency to be responsible for bringing together the coalition, for initiating the planning process, and for identifying what needs to be done and by whom. It simplifies the process if a lead agency can be designated at the outset. As an alternative to a designated lead agency, some communities have specific planning agencies, funded by United Way, which can help your coalition to develop plans and facilitate the planning process.

An ideal lead agency:

• Has skilled staff, or hires additional staff, who can be assigned to the task of conducting the background work, planning meetings and the needs assessment, and join in developing and implementing strategies;

• Includes representatives from both the public and private sectors;

• Is in a position to receive and allocate funds from both public and private sources. A mayoralty appointed commission might provide a good model as long as the governing board is broadly representative;

• Has the support of the city and state government (as appropriate);

• Has the technical expertise, in-house or through subcontract, to organize data gathering, design survey instruments, produce maps, conduct analysis, and prepare preliminary reports;

• Is acceptable to the community, and demonstrates sensitivity to the needs of disadvantaged families;

• Plays the lead in reviewing preliminary plans, and facilitating a consensus-building process;

- Serves as a liaison to the media, educates media representatives about the purpose of the community plan, and convinces media decision-makers to play an active role in its implementation.

The board (appointed or elected) must monitor the efforts of the lead agency, and assure that members of the coalition continue to play an active role in the planning and implementation phases.

The Role of a Lead Agency

Two major functions of the lead agency are: selecting an appropriate decision-making body, and doing the staff work for the detailed plan. While the lead agency should have the technical expertise to organize data gathering, design survey instruments, prepare preliminary reports, and so on, it is essential that other coalition members have an active role in the planning process.

Once the preliminary plan is completed, the lead agency will be responsible for a lengthy and often difficult review process. To arrive at consensus on the plan will require patience and skill, and the flexibility to incorporate changes resulting from this review process. Techniques have been developed that may be helpful in identifying alternative solutions, in resolving what the coalition's priorities will be, and in developing the necessary steps for implementing a plan of action. (See Appendix 4–2 for an example.)

When a plan has been agreed upon, implementation can get under way. The lead agency may be responsible for receiving grants, allocating funds to designated agencies, establishing referral mechanisms, arranging for evaluation and monitoring, organizing training and technical assistance, and in some cases, actually providing services.

If the lead agency is incorporated as a free-standing agency, and acts as a funding umbrella (receiving grants and allocating funds), one important function will be that of grants management. This calls for attention to accounting systems and uniform data collection — which is also important for monitoring and evaluation. The lead agency can assist local constituent agencies with their own fund raising, an effort that is greatly enhanced by documentation of program activities. The lead agency can expedite availability of training on fund-raising and other topics by serving as a community-wide resource for in-service training and workshops, and by bringing consultants and experts into the community for specific tasks.

In some communities, the community-wide plan may lead to development of a system of centralized case management. Because such a system involves many different considerations (pregnancy prevention, school retention, and job preparation), there may be no single appropriate agency to operate the system. In this case, the lead agency may take on this task, hiring, training, and supervising case managers, and placing them in the appropriate settings, such as schools and/or community centers.

Finally, the lead agency must be capable of relating to state administrative and policy entities. Much of the funding for sex and family life education, school-based clinics, school drop-out prevention, counseling, and other programs derives from state funding sources such as departments of maternal and child health, Medicaid, education, mental health, and special line items for specific services. (See Chapter 3.) Family planning clinics depend primarily on federal grants such as Title X, although most of those grants are administered and controlled by state agencies (typically the health department). Many states have pregnancy prevention task forces or are developing "youth-at-risk" initiatives that will produce funding for local pregnancy prevention programs, particularly demonstration projects, such as the comprehensive multi-service programs in New Jersey, and school drop-out prevention initiatives (Koshel, 1989).

The Role of the Coordinator

The crucial "glue" that makes community-wide efforts succeed is a dedicated coordinator. This individual is most often housed administratively within the lead agency and is responsible both to the lead agency and to the steering committee or board of directors. He or she must be technically competent, politically savvy, and strong in interpersonal relationships. Much of this person's effort will be in coordinating the efforts of other organizations, many of which will have to cross naturally occurring territorial lines. This is a job that requires an energetic and committed individual, who must also know how to delegate responsibility in an effective manner.

Making Coalition Meetings Work

Appendix 4–1 provides additional details on how to plan and conduct coalition meetings. Some ingredients of a successful meeting are listed below.

- Hold coalition meetings at a time when both professionals and other interested members can attend.

- Have agendas easily available and have a sign-in sheet with names and addresses for future mailings.

- Encourage key people to attend meetings by maintaining close follow-ups, including mailings and phone calls to confirm attendance.

- At the end of the meeting, review assignments, holding specific individuals and agencies responsible for completing specific tasks.

Facing Controversy

A number of alternative approaches are explored when communities search for solutions to the problem of adolescent pregnancy. Often tension exists surrounding these different courses of action. In some of the most successful cases, conflicts have been resolved by the inclusion of opposing groups in the data-gathering and planning process. This effort can result in the creation of a truly community-wide plan for the prevention of adolescent pregnancy.

Along the full continuum of interventions, different agencies and organizations may discover many areas of philosophical agreement, and other areas where there is no agreement. For a successful example of community negotiation, see the one cited on page 85; a planning group for one school-based health clinic reached a consensus that students who were pregnant would have the option of being referred to different agencies where they could receive counseling for each of the available options, including abortion, prenatal care to maintain the pregnancy, and adoption.

Involving the community can also offset the fears and feelings of powerlessness that may lead to opposition. Fear of controversy can pose a serious challenge to your efforts. A study conducted for the Centers for Disease Control reported that fear of opposition or controversy was the most common reason that school boards and administrators did not initiate, expand, or support sex education in schools. More important, however, the study found that in most communities only 1% of residents are irrevocably, opposed to sex education (Scales, 1982). This research also documented that communities that were most successful in implementing programs had developed specific strategies to promote community involvement and support.

After You Are Organized

Now that you have begun to organize your coalition around the process of developing a community-wide adolescent pregnancy prevention effort, you are ready to proceed with the next steps. A timetable must be generated and communicated to all coalition members. Allot at least a year for the planning and community development process, and for the search for any necessary additional funding. Program planning can be thought of as a cyclical process involving continuous monitoring and adjustment of the program to meet the needs of the target population. The five key steps in the cycle of program development are:

1. Assess community needs

2. Define goals and objectives

3. Design the intervention

4. Implement the intervention

5. Assess the effect of the intervention

This process assures that feedback about your community's needs is constantly being utilized in the program planning process. (See chart 4-3)

Chart 4-3

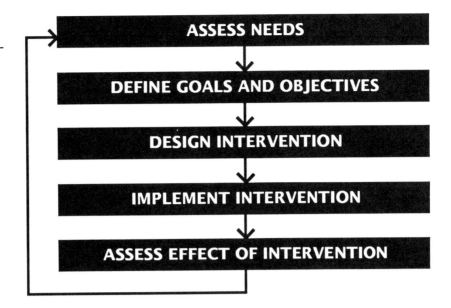

The first step in the planning process addresses the magnitude and intensity of the problem of teenage pregnancy in your community. This also involves evaluating the current delivery system for pregnancy prevention services, as well as the potential of local agencies to offer new or additional services. Most communities can come up with a reasonable estimate of unmet need: the difference between the ideal for that community as exemplified by locally agreed upon standards, and what actually exists. If all the necessary programs and facilities are in place, the primary task for the lead agency is coordination. If, on the other hand, the community has service gaps, the primary task may also include program planning and fundraising.

Close monitoring of the changes that occur in a community is an ongoing process, and one necessary for effective program planning. Information you gain from these observations will play an important part in your continuing efforts to assess the needs of your community, and to fine-tune your program. The remainder of this book will outline the details of each step of the program planning process.

Establishing a Set of Community Standards – How to Create Consensus

Before you are ready to implement your plan, you will need to develop a set of standards for service delivery, using group process and consensus-building exercises (see Appendix 4-3 for a step by step guide to this process).

This set of standards will help planners make decisions on where to place the community's resources, and provide a yardstick against which your coalition can measure how well the community is meeting the needs of its youthful population.

The following standards, based on the experience of our model community, Anytown, are suggested as a guideline for communities. They represent what could be the overall goals of the community-wide effort, and should reflect the values of that community.

Sample Standards
for Program
Development:
Potential Roles
of Community
Agencies in
Adolescent
Pregnancy
Prevention

These standards are built around a common set of assumptions that Anytown's Adolescent Pregnancy Prevention has adopted.

All teenagers need:

- Strong family relationships and guidance.

- Enhancement of self-esteem, goal development, and decision-making skills.

- Positive role models, including balanced media role models.

- Family life education that emphasizes the benefits of delaying the start of sexual intercourse, while recognizing the need for knowledge regarding all methods of birth control available to adolescents.

- Access to comprehensive health care (including general physical care, information on adolescent development, reproductive health care information, and counseling about abstinence, contraception, abortion, and adoption) and the provision of appropriate services.

- Educational training to prepare young people for the workplace and for their roles as parents.

- Job training and employment opportunities.

- Recognition of the importance of, and shared responsibility for, sexual activity, reproduction, and parenting.

In addition, we believe:

- Community involvement with, and investment in, young people is vital to the overall health of the community.

- Implementation of the community-wide plan requires active partnerships and collaboration among teenagers, parents, religious organizations, local communities, state and federal agencies, and nongovernmental organizations. All steps taken to implement the plan's strategies and standards must reflect the community's cultural and ethnic diversity.

- Prevention of teenage pregnancy is a key issue to be addressed from early years through adolescence.

- Economic barriers to accessible and comprehensive services (health, education, job training, etc.) must be reduced, if not eliminated.

- Every young person should have access to a responsible adult for guidance and support.

Community and
Agency Standards

Family and Schools

- Social institutions (families, daycare centers, schools, and community organizations involved with youths) should provide each child with a safe environment that fosters a sense of responsibility; that establishes rules, parameters, rewards, positive reinforcement, and effective communication; and that affirms the child through love.

- Schools, which have great impact on a child's life potential, should provide a supportive environment, and effective teaching and counseling should provide students with a personal assessment that allows them to set high goals.

- Parenting education, including ways to encourage development of childrearing skills, should begin with pregnancy and be reinforced throughout the child's developmental phases.

- Schools should provide young parents with additional skill-building in interpersonal relations, social skills, and success-oriented experiences, including literacy.

- Parents of teenagers should be actively involved in health education, including family life education, through schools and agencies. Parents should be encouraged to take an active part in the education of their children, and to support their children in career planning.

- Schools should provide job-related learning opportunities and meaningful extracurricular activities that are community-based, accessible, and neighborhood-centered. Existing programs, such as sports facilities, clubs, nonprofit organizations, and businesses should work with schools to establish stable and enriching experiences, using the school site.

- By high school graduation, all teenagers should have received a comprehensive K–12 health education program, including family life education.

- Uniform core standards should be established for both the content and the qualifications of those teaching health education. While the core curriculum can be integrated into relevant courses, such as biology or life science, family life education topics can also be woven into social sciences and English in order to reinforce the teaching.

- Peer education and peer counseling should be established, with teen expert panels available for presentations, and courses for teenage parents provided to supplement the core curriculum.

- One teacher at each school should be responsible for integrating health education curricula.

- School systems should arrange and pay for teacher in-service training and supervision in family life education.

- All school "gatekeepers" (e.g. principals, vice-principals, counselors, school nurses, and other administrative staff) should receive orientation in dealing with sexuality issues.

Health Providers

The goal should be to establish accessible, available, affordable, comprehensive, and coordinated health care for adolescents through the network of health providers in the community, including services that:

- Are flexible in their hours of availability, and geared to after-school appointments,

- Emphasize continuity of care, rather than a crisis focus and episodic care,

- Are adequately funded in order to provide care for teenagers who are un-insured or under-insured,

- Assure confidentiality of care as provided by law,

- Provide referral and follow-up to other services for adolescents as appropriate,

- Provide full psychosocial histories, including histories of risk-taking behaviors, as part of the comprehensive assessment and treatment services provided,

- Access a coordinated system of care for youth, including primary care, mental health services, substance abuse services, family planning education and care, health education, stress management, and referrals for other community-based agencies and services, as appropriate,

- Inform adolescents of available health services in their communities and teach them how to be effective health consumers,

- Provide a well-publicized central phone number where adolescents' questions can be answered, and where they can receive information and referrals for health programs as appropriate,

- Link to school and other community sites either through the co-location of a health professional for a minimum of four hours per week, and/or through the in-service training of school and agency personnel to refer adolescents to the appropriate community health programs,

- Establish health care standards for each provider: for example, guidelines as to appropriate staffing, medical coverage, documentation, emergency back-up system, follow-up of referrals, etc.

Youth-serving Agencies

- Develop interagency cooperation between schools and community agencies concerned with youth issues, and encourage the use of the school site or other centrally located site to co-locate services. This may include expansion of enriching extracurricular activities that occur at the school site, as well as opportunities to learn about the variety of community resources available to youths.

- Develop mentoring programs and job shadowing (exposure to on-site work experiences) for youths, to expose them to the world of work. These might include volunteer, apprenticeship and paid job opportunities, depending on the levels of the students.

- Provide training in job seeking, interview skills, resumé development, and employers' expectations. Assist youths in identifying potential work experiences.

- Expand efforts to reach dropouts, and provide them with assistance to pursue alternative routes for earning a high school diploma and educational and training opportunities beyond high school.

- Sponsor and implement programs that help teenagers help each other. These might teach communication skills, encourage responsible decision making, encourage peer counseling, support community involvement and teenage responsibility, and reward success. Include the creation of support and self-help groups conducted through the auspices of community agencies.

- Increase public awareness of the availability of community agencies through media coverage and the use of a centralized information and referral system.

- Ensure that interagency efforts are broad-based in order to provide teenagers with opportunities for their future, including education, employment training, housing, and recreation.

Summary

The coalition should work towards establishing a comprehensive array of goals against which the community can begin to assess the progress they have made. Many of these standards will emerge from the needs assessment process, which will document where the gaps exist in the community. In setting standards, coalition members may want to consider what the ideal situation for youth living in the community would be, and strive over time to work on meeting these ideals. It is also important, however, to consider what resources are available, and what aspects of these standards can be met through currently available services and programs. The coalition may also need to consider establishing priorities within these standards. For example, they may consider it a priority to develop more comprehensive family life education before focusing on strengthening interagency collaboration, or they may see that both can be accomplished simultaneously by having schools work closer with health and social agencies in implementing a curriculum and referral program. As a means of ensuring clarity of purpose, it is important to develop a comprehensive array of standards which relate to each of the major components of the plan and the community. The coalition must also consider whether any sanctions need to be implemented (e.g. funding diminished if goals are not met within an agreed upon time framework).

When a coalition begins to take shape in a community, the first steps for the initial members are formulation of a broad-based community organization with representation from a wide range of agencies, and designation of a lead agency, a board of directors or steering committee, and a coordinator. Representation on the coalition and the board should reflect the community in terms of sex, race/ethnicity, and socioeconomic background, and both the coalition and its board should include a comprehensive and diverse selection of key groups and agencies in the community. The board and the lead agency can work together to implement the goals and objectives of the coalition. The board can provide the direction, and the lead agency can do the staff work. The coordinator is the fourth key ingredient — after the coalition, the board, and the lead agency. Selection of this individual should be based on his or her estimated ability to work successfully with the entire range of agencies in the coalition, and to handle important relationships with other community and political groups.

All coalition members must maintain an active role in the planning process if the endeavor is to be a success. Their full involvement can help to head off controversy and conflict during the crucial process of conducting the needs assessment, developing an implementation plan, and adopting the courses of action deemed necessary to adequately address the community's problems.

Appendix 4-1

The Initial Planning Meeting

*A*ssuming that there is an individual or small group of individuals initiating the coalition building process, there are some important tasks to accomplish prior to as well as during the initial planning meeting. Be sure that adequate time is devoted to planning the very first meeting as it will help establish the tone of the work that will be accomplished through the coalition. Planning worksheets are included in this appendix, while "A Coalition Building Checklist," adapted from a manual on the art of coalition building (Brown, 1981) is included in Appendix 4-2. The questions listed on that checklist may also be helpful in developing agenda items for the meeting(s). An additional guide, "Building and Maintaining Effective Coalitions," part of the "How-To Guides on Community Health Promotion," produced by the Stanford Health Promotion Resource Center, is also a helpful resource. (See General Resource Directory, page 273.)

Before the Meeting

1. Begin considering what a coalition "mission" statement should consist of. For example, the Dallas Coalition on Adolescent Pregnancy has as its mission statement, "to systematically involve all segments of the community in reducing school-age pregnancy by providing improved health, education, and social services to adolescents." This mission statement can be expanded during the first meeting as the purpose and goals of the coalition are discussed. It is important to establish realistic expectations, as well as a feasible timeline.

2. Prepare a draft outline of a committee structure that can be discussed as plans are made for future meetings and activities.

3. Formulate options for developing an operating structure (refer to discussion of the lead agency, pp. 87-89). If there is already an obvious choice for lead agency, such as United Way, mayor's office, or health planning agency, this should be made clear. If there is no obvious choice, outline the options.

4. If possible, recruit a respected community leader to issue the invitation to join the coalition.

5. Follow up on all invitations, and make sure that the turnout at the first meeting is representative and broad.

6. Decide whether you want to go public from the outset, and if so use the media to announce the meeting. In most instances, the coalition meeting should be as inclusive and public as possible.

Conducting the Meeting

1. Have agendas readily available and have a sign-in sheet to document who was present, and to correct names and addresses for future mailings. Participants should introduce themselves, perhaps sharing with the group their interest in the area of adolescent pregnancy and pregnancy prevention. The meeting should be chaired by an effective group facilitator who is seen as a neutral party.

2. Discuss and revise the mission statement as necessary to reflect the goals of the group. If diverse groups are to come together to solve a problem, they must have a common definition of the problem. Many efforts at collaboration dissolve into fierce turf battles months later because this necessary first step is overlooked in the rush to move ahead (Dunkle, 1988).

   Sharing a common vision is a unifying principal of coalition building and an essential ingredient of community ownership of the program, and it is for this reason that the coalition may want to explore the idea of selecting a neutral facilitator to assist in developing goals and objectives. Sometimes using a neutral organization to build strong coalitions of powerful participants can be effective, especially when the issues are controversial and agency funds are at stake (Dunkle, 1988). After the mission statement is approved, the following are questions for discussion:

   a. What objective do you hope to accomplish through this community-wide effort?

   b. Is there a critical mass of individuals, agencies, organizations, etc. who are committed to developing a community-wide strategy? How much and what kind of support can be expected from these potential participants?

   c. What resources exist? What funds, personnel, volunteer support, and other help are or might be available?

   d. What barriers to developing a community-wide strategy exist? What policy or regulatory barriers, such as state regulations, might act to block the integration of various types of services? What administrative issues and structures exist, such as insurance or liability or permission requirements? What steps are necessary to circumvent any identified barriers to community-wide efforts?

e. What is the current level of working relationships among schools and other community agencies? What collaborative relationships are already in place?

3. By the end of the meeting, make assignments and hold individuals or agencies responsible for fulfilling specific requirements for the next meeting.

4. Designate support staff to assist the coordinator in keeping and mailing minutes. Future mailings should include a copy of the minutes of the meeting as well as an agenda for the next meeting.

5. Establish a regular meeting schedule and a convenient site. This will help assure continuity and coordination. Hold coalition meetings at a time when both professionals and other interested members can attend.

6. If key policymakers from all the agencies serving youth have not attended this first meeting, it is important to follow up to ensure their involvement. These individuals are key to ensuring nonduplication of services and cooperative planning and programming.

7. Begin planning specific steps for the next coalition meetings. Determine what tasks will be accomplished during future meetings and what tasks will require additional background work.

Your meeting will depend somewhat upon the composition of the group, and members' knowledge of the consequences of adolescent pregnancy in your community. If it is appropriate, provide attendees with a short background paper on the issue. A group discussion of the current impact of adolescent pregnancy on the different agencies can also facilitate the development of a shared mission statement.

Use brainstorming and group consensus techniques (Appendix 4-3) to develop the mission statement, goals, and objectives. If the group is large, you may plan to break into smaller groups to make the process more workable. Conclusions and issues discussed in the smaller groups may then be shared with the larger group.

Plan how you will take care of meeting logistics to ensure everything runs smoothly. Arrange for work areas for both small and large group activities. Provide writing materials for use during the group discussion and plan how you will handle registration, name tags, and refreshments.

Ideally a first meeting should last two to three hours. Some groups prefer to hold a brief meeting to plan a longer retreat in which coalition members spend an entire day together.

Suggested Agenda

The following is a suggested agenda for a first meeting.

AGENDA
Establishing a Coalition for Developing Community-wide Strategies for Adolescent Pregnancy Prevention

I. Introductions (initial members of the coalition, agency representatives, guests)

II. Purpose of meeting and the reason to develop a coalition: Why is adolescent pregnancy prevention a needed focus in our community?

III. Potential Roles of the Coalition

    a. Mission

    b. Goals

    c. Objectives

IV. Discuss Steps to be Taken in the Development of a Community-wide Strategic Plan

    a. Planning the needs assessment

    b. Developing a community plan based upon the findings of the needs assessment and available resources

    c. Implementation of the plan

    d. Evaluation of the program

V. Next Steps and Planning of Future Meetings

Worksheets

The following worksheets are included to help you plan the first meeting of the coalition (Appendix 4-1), as well as to consider what the role and function of the coalition will be in your community (Appendix 4-2).

Worksheet 4-1

Worksheet: Planning for the First Meeting

1. Proposed mission statement:_____

   _____

   _____

   _____

2. Outline of committee structure (description or diagram):

3. Lead agency:_____

   Coordinator:_____

4. Agenda Items:_____

   _____

   _____

   _____

5. List of invited agencies, community leaders, and members of the media:

Name:	Affiliation:	Attending: Yes	No
1.			
2.			
3.			
4.			
5.			
6.			
7.			
8.			
9.			
10.			
11.			
12.			
13.			
14.			
15.			
16.			
17.			
18.			
19.			
20.			

Appendix 4-2

A Coalition-building Checklist

Worksheet 4-2

_U_se the following questions to help guide your coalition-building efforts. These items have been adapted from a manual on the art of coalition building (Brown 1981).

Getting Started

1. Has at least one of these catalysts generated interest in forming a coalition:

   - a significantly committed individual ___ Yes ___ No

   - a disturbing or dramatic event ___ Yes ___ No

   - detailed, timely information about the issue. ___ Yes ___ No

2. Will a coalition help potential members achieve goals they cannot achieve alone? ___ Yes ___ No

3. Is each potential member organization committed to working on the issue? ___ Yes ___ No

4. Are there formal leadership links between potential coalition members? ___ Yes ___ No

Building a Constituency

1. Have any groups already done work on the issue? ___ Yes ___ No

2. Is it known which groups will benefit from action on the issue? ___ Yes ___ No

3. Is there an outline of separate strategies to attract each group to join the coalition? ___ Yes ___ No

4. Is there a list of resources (e.g. staff time, money, publicity) expected from each member organization?   ___ Yes ___ No

5. Do the by-laws of each member group permit participation in the work of the coalition?   ___ Yes ___ No

6. Does the person representing each organization have the power to act on behalf of that organization?   ___ Yes ___ No

7. Will certain organizations need incentives to join?   ___ Yes ___ No

Joining a Coalition: What Groups Should Consider

1. Will the member organization gain visibility?   ___ Yes ___ No

2. Will membership potential be increased?   ___ Yes ___ No

3. Will links be created with other important organizations?   ___ Yes ___ No

4. Does the potential member have the resources to contribute:

• staff time   ___ Yes ___ No

• money   ___ Yes ___ No

• office space   ___ Yes ___ No

• new allies   ___ Yes ___ No

• research capabilities   ___ Yes ___ No

• a better reputation in the community   ___ Yes ___ No

• media and press coverage   ___ Yes ___ No

• a broader constituency   ___ Yes ___ No

5. Is there comparability between the organization's philosophy and the philosophy of the coalition?   ___ Yes ___ No

Mapping Out Coalition Strategy

1. Will invitations to join the coalition be extended to concerned organizations early enough for them to contribute to the formulation of strategy?   ___ Yes ___ No

2. Have the positions of groups that may be reluctant to join ___ Yes ___ No
the coalition been carefully checked to see if differences
of opinion can be bridged?

3. Is there an arrangement for groups that might come to the coa- ___ Yes ___ No
lition with other urgent issues to find a forum for those issues?

4. Is there an agreement to focus on the key issue around ___ Yes ___ No
which the coalition was formed, and to refrain from adding
other issues that may be important to other member groups?

5. Have controversial positions on which there is no ___ Yes ___ No
consensus been put into non-binding statements, to avoid
trying to force an agreement?

*Coalition
Leadership*

1. Has each member been approached by the leader in order ___ Yes ___ No
to build a one-to-one relationship?

2. Is the leader able to elicit every member's thinking, to ___ Yes ___ No
consult widely among members, and then draw the thinking
into a concrete program?

3. Can the leader help the coalition move forward after ___ Yes ___ No
defeats and, in times of discouragement, recognize the
successes it has achieved?

4. Have one or more replacements been selected for ___ Yes ___ No
leadership training?

5. Is the leader willing to disband the coalition when it has
outlived its usefulness? ___ Yes ___ No

*The Coalition's
Internal Functions*

Staff

1. Is it clear which member organizations will contribute ___ Yes ___ No
staff or where the staff will come from?

2. Is there an explicit agreement about the role of staff in ___ Yes ___ No
coalition decisions?

Decision Making

1. Has the coalition decided who will speak for it in public? ___ Yes ___ No

2. Have any of these procedures been agreed upon for making coalition decisions?

- consensus   ___ Yes ___ No

- democratic voting   ___ Yes ___ No

- organizational vetoes   ___ Yes ___ No

- other   ___ Yes ___ No

Fundraising and Maintaining Commitment

1. Does the coalition have a procedure that avoids   ___ Yes ___ No
competition for funding among member organizations?

2. Does the coalition leadership allow multiple levels of   ___ Yes ___ No
commitment on the part of member organizations?

Appendix 4-3

Decision-making Approaches for Your Board and Coalition

*G*round rules for group discussion and decision-making become imperative as your coalition and its steering committee (board of directors) develop. Given the potential controversy of some key decisions that will be made by the group, it is important to establish a process by which the group can select among alternatives.

There are three factors to consider when deciding upon this process (Burghardt, 1982):

1. The size and make-up of the group

2. The percentage of new people attending

3. The degree and intensity of differences among attendees

If your coalition is small in size and homogeneous in its attitudes, an informal discussion format can be used. However, if you have a variety of attitudes and desired approaches to the problem, a more formal method such as Robert's Rules of Order may be more appropriate. While this method does not seem relaxed, it may lead to more order and democratic functioning during meetings, and prevent discussion from wandering without resolution.

There are many approaches to decision-making, and each has certain consequences for the way your group will function. The following decision-making methods are readily identifiable, though not always desirable (Kitzi, 1986):

1. *Decision by Lack of Response:* Someone suggests an idea and nobody responds;

another idea is suggested. The group has passively decided to bypass the first idea, and not to adopt it.

2. *Decision by Authority Rule:* The chairperson, or someone with authority, makes decisions. The group can generate ideas, but the chairperson or other person makes all final decisions. This approach may produce a minimum amount of group involvement, and diminish the quality of the implementation of the decision.

3. *Decision by Minority:* Two or three members of the group press for a quick decision before opposition can build. This can produce feelings that the decision was railroaded: the assumption that silence means consent is not necessarily true. Often those feeling left out of the decision-making process will not help (and may hinder) implementation of any decision reached in this manner.

4. *Decision by Majority Rule:* Decisions are made by voting and/or polling after some discussion. If the majority is in favor, the majority vote is accepted as a decision. Problems may arise from this method when a member holding a minority position feels that there was insufficient time for discussion. The meeting facilitator must be sure to allow adequate time for discussion from a variety of viewpoints. A split in the group may be created with the "losers" looking for a way to "win" next time.

5. *Decision by Consensus:* This is one of the most time-consuming methods for problem solving in groups since it is a process for making full use of group members. It is also an approach for exposing and exploring conflicting viewpoints before reaching a decision (Heimovide and Kitzi, 1986).

Clearly the first three decision-making approaches will conflict with the development of a strong coalition, while decision by majority rule (with adequate discussion) and consensus will help to build and strengthen efforts to build trust among coalition members.

Consensus

Consensus is not the same as unanimity – it is the arrival at a decision that each member can accept. Sufficient open discussion is encouraged so that everyone has a fair chance to influence a decision. Someone then tests to find the "sense of the group," avoiding a formal vote. If after full discussion of various viewpoints, there is a clear course of action to which most members can subscribe, consensus exists. This requires the exploration of a variety of alternatives and the rationale for these alternatives. A wide range of opinions and information usually gives the group a chance to develop a more creative and adequate solution that is acceptable to the group.

There are also drawbacks to adopting decision-making by consensus. Discussions may go on at such length that people will agree so that they can close the meeting. As with the majority vote, it is likely that some individuals may not be totally satisfied with the decision, feeling they have had to sacrifice some of their beliefs so that action can be taken (Burghardt, 1982).

An alternative approach, the nominal group process, shows one approach for gaining group consensus in establishing group priorities.

Nominal Group Process

The nominal group technique incorporates planned brainstorming techniques (Kitzi, 1986), which are particularly helpful in identifying alternative methods of establishing priorities. The nominal group process is usually conducted by a group facilitator or leader with groups of (ideally) between five and nine persons. It can be incorporated in a number of group tasks, such as program planning or exploration of roadblocks to progress, as well as in surfacing alternative solutions. The process, approximately one hour in length, should be followed consistently in order to achieve maximum benefit. This technique strengthens the investment of the group in developing the necessary steps for implementing a plan. Its advantage over open discussion is that it encourages maximum and equal individual participation in the generation and judgement of solutions, without allowing the status or special expertise of some members to overly influence the group's choice. It is a carefully structured procedure that requires individuals to privately list ideas, clarify those ideas, and rank them to produce a picture of the group's judgement.

As "doers," our usual behavior is to rush prematurely into action on the first or second solution that occurs to us. This method, by contrast, seeks to surface the best creative thinking of each individual in the group, to produce a full list of alternatives, and to discover which solution is most representative of the group's thinking (Kitzi, 1986).

Steps in the Nominal Group Process

1. *Statement of the Problem:* The problem should be clearly stated so that each member of the group may quickly grasp the problem and contribute his/her ideas. After the problem statement has been developed, it is desirable to consider a number of alternative solutions before moving to planning actions and strategies.

   It is important for the leader to explain the exercise and set the stage for the fact that the success of the process is dependent on all members sharing their personal insights. Furthermore, each person's contribution will have equal weight.

2. *Silent Individual Listing of Ideas in Writing:* Each group member lists alternative strategies for reaching the goal identified by the coalition. Encourage participants to use short phrases and to avoid communication with other group members during this step. This process is in sharp contrast to regular brainstorming, in which ideas are contributed as rapidly as possible and recorded on chart pad or chalk board. Allocate approximately 15 minutes for this step.

3. *Round Robin Recording of Ideas:* Ideas are listed on a flip chart with each group

member quickly offering one of his or her ideas per turn. The facilitator should number the ideas as they are written for later reference. Continue rounds of listing single ideas from each person until all ideas are listed. There should be no attempt to evaluate or pass judgement on an idea. Members of the group are urged to show consideration for their fellow members so that all ideas get recorded. New ideas that occur to members during the process can also be added to the list in turn.

The purpose of this step is to elicit as many ideas as possible in a brief period of time. Generating one idea at a time ensures that all ideas will be listed, and that they will be less personally identified than would happen if a cluster of ideas were to be given by each individual in turn.

4. *Serial Discussion of Ideas for Clarification*: Respondents discuss each idea in turn. With questions, clarifications, agreement, disagreement, or any statement related to the suggested solution, the group moves from item to item, discussing each briefly. Group members are encouraged to avoid arguing or lobbying for any one idea in particular. The focus is kept on the clarification of solutions listed. Without attempting an evaluation, members of the group can combine ideas where appropriate, subsume others under major headings, and weed out duplicate ideas.

5. *Ranking Alternative Solutions:* The ranking procedure allows the group to develop a clear, collective picture of their priority rankings of suggested solutions . It allows individual members to make independent decisions that will be weighted equally. To do this each participant will:

- Select the five highest priority solutions from the total list of ideas posted. Then write each of those solutions on a separate index card, placing the list number of the item on the top left hand corner.

- Spread out all the cards and decide which rates the highest priority, marking that card with a #5 in the lower right hand corner, and underlining the number. That index card is turned over and the remaining four cards are reviewed. Select the least important item and write a #1 in the right hand lower corner, and underline the number.

- Choose the most important of the three remaining cards, and mark it with a #4 in lower right corner, underlining the number. Then choose the least important of the remaining two items and mark it #2 in the lower right corner. Mark the remaining card #3 in lower right corner.

The leader collects the cards to protect the anonymity of votes and proceeds to record all rankings in the margin beside each item listed, on the flip chart or on a separate numbered tally sheet.

Example: Voting Tally Sheet

Item from Round Robin	Rank Order Scores of Group
1	3-2-3-1
2	2-3-3-4-2
3	2-1-1-1-2-1
4	5-4-5-5-4
5	4-4-3-5-5

You can repeat the process of ranking the items until the group members reach agreement on major strategies and establish their priorities. Through this process the group casts aside ideas that are not germane to the problem and those found impractical or impossible to deal with.

6. *Action Stage:* Before you can act on the priority items, it is important to assess both potential barriers and implementation resources available. Developing a plan for implementing the chosen solutions may require a variety of simultaneous strategies.

Among the many questions to resolve are:

a. Who else should be working on this project apart from the agency or coalition?

b. Where do we begin?

c. How do we begin?

d. Who will do what to get us started?

e. When do we start?

Chapter 5

Needs Assessment and Data Collection

---

*C*onducting a community-based needs assessment is a vital step in designing an effective community-wide adolescent pregnancy prevention program. The resulting report should describe gaps in services, potential models and programs that will help meet (or close) identified gaps, and the types of approaches that may be most successful in your community. The needs assessment helps establish both community requirements and potential resources. It is a crucial step in planning a coordinated effort, both in communities where there are already many youth-oriented programs and in those that have few such efforts underway. If a community-based program has no existing adolescent pregnancy prevention component, the needs assessment process will help delineate the program's role. The document will show how many adolescent pregnancy prevention efforts already exist within the community, and identify additional efforts that are needed. Needs assessments may include surveys of programs and community organizations as well as individuals who may be affected by the problem, or who are at risk (e.g., youth, parents).

A needs assessment is a means to an end, not an end in itself. The nature of the problem, the resources that are available, and the variety of perceptions and attitudes exhibited toward resolving these problems will vary greatly among communities. In all cases, however, conducting a needs assessment will help establish goals, define tasks, and fix responsibilities for accomplishing the desired goals, including funding and evaluation. Conducting a needs assessment in the area of prevention can be particularly challenging, since programs and policies in this arena have usually not been as clearly delineated as are efforts geared to serving adolescents who are either pregnant or already parents.

What is a Needs Assessment?

The term "needs assessment" means different things to different people. Generally, it goes beyond simple documentation of need (how many sexually active teens there are in the community who are at risk of unintended pregnancy, etc.) to documentation of *unmet* needs. For example, an assessment might establish how many teens at risk do *not* have access to prevention programs. On an issue as sensitive as adolescent pregnancy, assessment sometimes goes further than defining unmet needs and addresses the potential for action — perceptions of problems; priority of problem; climate for action; potential for development; and commitment of new resources.

A needs assessment will help to:

• Determine the extent of the problem with estimates of need and unmet need,

• Evaluate community efforts to prevent teenage pregnancy, by documenting the baseline problem and current community activities,

• Outline the way the problem is perceived by young people, service providers, public officials (elected and appointed), and other community members,

• Evaluate resources available to address problems, including programs already in place, and funding sources,

• Assess the environment for development of new resources,

• Assess the climate for collaboration, for allocation of new resources, and/or interest in developing adolescent pregnancy prevention components in existing or new programs.

Why Do a Community-wide Needs Assessment?

Frequently, a community will attempt to implement model programs conducted in other communities without first determining if the needs of the communities are similar, or how such a model program will fit into their community's own overall network of services. Highly publicized programs sometimes produce a bandwagon effect, but their replication can lead to failure unless all the key ingredients originally available are in place. Tailoring programs and activities to local needs and resources requires a thorough assessment of your particular community. A superficial knowledge of community problems and concerns will usually result in simplistic solutions that rarely work.

There are additional advantages to doing a community needs assessment:

• It is a way to develop or reinforce contacts with public officials and professionals concerned with the issue of adolescent pregnancy prevention.

• It paves the way for advocating the issue with public officials.

- If done carefully, it demonstrates your group's interest in and dedication to your community prior to project development.

- It helps identify community organizations that may be interested in working collaboratively to develop and implement programs, and therefore reduces duplication of service.

- It provides the objective documentation necessary to negotiate arrangements among agencies, helping to overcome existing constraints and possible turf issues.

- It allows those individuals most involved in, or touched by, the issue of adolescent pregnancy to define the problem as they perceive it, thus making an initial investment toward creating a solution.

- It provides the documentation of needs that is absolutely essential when applying for funds and other support.

- It provides an opportunity to actively involve parents and youths in data-gathering and interviewing.

- It provides a database, or baseline, against which resulting programs can be evaluated for effectiveness.

- It helps to educate a group and a community on the issue, regardless of followup efforts and activities.

Interorganizational Relationships

In addition to finding the various community organizations already working with youths, it is important to assess working relationships (formal and informal) between agencies. Relationships that are already established may provide ready-made strategic alliances that can create innovative programs.

Given the potential difficulty of developing and attracting new funding into a community, it is important that the needs assessment process also provide the opportunity to assess funding sources already in place, to examine how those funds are being utilized, and to consider whether reallocation of funding is desirable and feasible. While direct reallocation of funding among organizations may not be possible, a redistribution of staff time may create new options for communities. In addition, as the definition of adolescent pregnancy prevention widens, all youth-serving agencies should be assessed for their current role (and the possible expansion of that role) in adolescent pregnancy prevention efforts. For example, a police department may have a youth activities league, or a college fraternity may initiate a mentoring program involving the development of sexual responsibility in addition to leadership skills.

Consider Your Goals

As you begin to plan the needs assessment process, it is imperative to consider what goals are guiding the effort. For example, if the reason for doing the assessment is to document that there is an adolescent pregnancy problem in your community, then much of the focus of the assessment will be on gathering data to document the extent of the problem, the kinds of services that are in place, and the gaps between the needs and the existing services, or the unmet need. You may also supplement these data with focus groups and youth surveys which can provide illustrative case histories and other descriptive data. As described later in this chapter, there are a great number of sources of data available to help you conduct your needs assessment. You can use a combination of these resources in doing your community study.

If your community is aware of the extent of the problem, but has not been able to arrive at a consensus on the solutions, the focus of your needs assessment will be on identification of the problems and barriers that stand in the way of consensus. If, on the other hand, your community appears to provide sufficient services, but the primary issue seems to be lack of coordination and involvement among schools and youth-serving agencies, then the focus of your assessment will be on identifying barriers to coordination – problems that schools and other youth-serving agencies encounter with adolescent pregnancy prevention efforts. Gauging where your community stands on the issue of developing a community-wide adolescent pregnancy prevention effort is a critical first step in developing a conceptual framework for your needs assessment.

A comprehensive needs assessment should also help you determine the extent to which the community is committed to pursuing particular goals (e.g., K-12 sex education). If commitment is not adequate, the needs assessment should provide you with a good understanding of why support is lacking and potential ways to overcome obstacles to change. Thus, a needs assessment can also be used as a strategic planning tool.

Needs assessment data can also be used to bridge information and communication gaps among service providers. If the needs assessment survey has been a multi-agency endeavor, the framework then exists for cooperative use of data to address community needs. When efficient service delivery is the issue (rather than territorial prerogatives or rivalry among agencies) cooperative planning may enable participating agencies to ameliorate the problem of limited financial resources.

What is the Target Community?

As a crucial first step you will need to define the actual parameters of the community for which a broad-based plan is being developed. Does the "community" refer to a state, county, or city, or does it encompass a smaller area? The community may also be defined by non-geographic parameters, including culture, language, and demographics (e.g. age, socio-economic status). Whatever the size of the community, it is critical to conduct an in-depth analysis of the extent of the problem by specific area, whether by health planning area, census tract, school district, or zip code. If the data are not specifically broken down by area, your capacity for developing priorities will be limited. Both the incidence of adolescent births and the extent that services are available and utilized in each of these designated areas must be studied as part of the needs assessment.

Ideally, one would like to be able to document the adolescent pregnancy rate in each area that comprises the target community. However, in order to calculate the pregnancy rate, one needs to document the incidence of births, miscarriages, and abortions. If abortion data are not readily available by community (and they rarely are), then birth rates have to be used as surrogate numbers to indicate the incidence of adolescent pregnancy (Appendix 5-1 provides a guide to assist you in calculating the birthrate for the community).

Other measures of need, such as the incidence of school dropout, can help you develop a fuller perspective of the problems young people face in your community. An even better indicator of adolescents at risk is the percentage of middle school adolescents behind their modal grade. Whatever indicators you choose, select a few measures that are available, and apply those measures as specifically as possible to the target population in order to establish the extent of the problem in the community.

Estimating Unmet Need

The estimate of unmet need is the most challenging to determine. In order to accomplish this task, you will need to develop an ideal standard of services, given the numbers and rates of adolescents in need. (See Chapter 4 for discussion of community standards.) The coalition may want to develop and build consensus on what this set of standards should consist of. The following are examples of standards a community might establish based on recommendations of the National Research Council's *Risking the Future* (1987) report:

- Every child should have access to K-12 sex education that includes birth control information, decision-making, problem-solving and communication skills, encouragement to delay the initiation of sexual activity, as well as birth control information and referrals.

- Every sexually active child should have access to contraception, and counseling on sexual responsibility.

- Every high-risk child (failing in school, lacking support at home, engaged in risk-taking behaviors) should have support from at least one adult, and should receive educational remediation, employment assistance, and health services.

Once guiding principles are established and agreed upon, the needs assessment can determine how well the standards are being met. For example, the needs assessment may document that while approximately 5,000 students are enrolled in K-12th grades, only 300 students are receiving family life education. Therefore, if family life education is established as a priority within the community-wide plan, the community will need to implement a K-12th grade curriculum, teacher training, and monitoring of the program. Different agencies may be available to help meet this standard; for example, the school system could be selected to be primarily responsible for implementation of the program, but could also receive assistance from other local agencies.

Getting Started

The first step in beginning the needs assessment process is to ask the following questions about your community:

1. In the areas of management, planning, and research, what are the knowledge and skill levels of those responsible for developing the community-wide plan? What is the focus for these individuals?

2. What resources are available to develop new strategies? Potential community resources include pooled funds from cooperating agencies, funds from government, private foundations, in-kind services, and volunteers.

3. What are public attitudes toward adolescent pregnancy prevention efforts?

Your needs assessment will have relatively little value unless: 1) capable individuals are available to analyze and follow through on the findings; 2) cooperation is available from such key potential delivery settings as the community's schools; and 3) the community is generally in favor of efforts in these areas.

The Scope of Your Assessment

A large-scale assessment is not always possible or necessary. The scope and depth of the needs assessment will depend on how much information is available, how current existing data are, attitudes in the community about the initiation of new programs or the reallocation of available resources, and how you plan to use the data collected.

The needs assessment should be broad enough to be "doable," without being so narrow in scope that it might fail to uncover a need for other, related programs. The community needs assessment process phase is an ideal time to adjust the goals of the program based on findings concerning documented need. That is, while your initial interest and commitment may lie in the area of adolescent pregnancy prevention, your investigation may document a need for other types of programs, such as drug prevention, employment training, etc., with a lesser, but still important component devoted to adolescent pregnancy prevention. By extending your assessment to encompass a broader array of youth problems and youth-serving agencies, you are responding to the need for a diverse set of strategies to expand life options for adolescents, as well as to provide accessible family planning care. Many young people are affected by a range of stresses and problems, and are often served concurrently by a variety of agencies.

Both the community assessment process and the strategies that emerge must respond to a multiplicity of problems.

The amount of time required to coordinate this broad approach is extensive, and this should be recognized at the outset. Considering potential time and resource limitations, it may be especially important for the lead agency to join with other professionals, organizations, or trained volunteers. In some cases you may wish to seek grant support for a staff member or consultant to coordinate and conduct the study. Some foundations have discretionary funding available that provides short-term support for the initial planning phase of program development. Many professional and business groups will provide free assistance to voluntary groups in developing and interpreting surveys. Local universities, colleges, advertising agencies, public relations firms, and political pollsters may contribute to your process, including assisting in collecting the information. For example, academic programs in public health, social work, sociology, psychology, education and marketing all may require community work. Other community agencies may be in the position to provide in-kind support (e.g., staff time, use of computer, etc.) to help move the assessment forward.

The depth and breadth of your assessment will depend upon the following factors:

- **What you already know.**
  You will need to determine what needs assessment information is available or has been previously collected. This enables you to focus on updating or adding to what has already been done. For example, in recent years, state and local health agencies, local chapters of the Junior League, and members of the General Federation of Women's Clubs have conducted independent surveys of their communities. It is important to research previous efforts, as many communities feel they have been "over-studied." They can point to a shelf full of reports that sit collecting dust because no steps were taken to plan and implement the recommended actions.

- **What information is needed immediately.**
  All components do not have to be undertaken simultaneously. If a primary purpose of the needs assessment is to get a community effort off the ground (generate urgency, set the stage for development of a coalition, etc.), then the first step could be limited to data collection. The coalition itself can advocate that the city fund and implement a services assessment or conduct a youth survey. The lead organization can also suggest that a comprehensive needs assessment be the first task for the coalition and use this as a team-building tool.

- **Resources available.**
  Commitment to conducting the assessment should match resources that are available, including knowledge, skills, and external resources. Your group may need to scale down the extent of the needs assessment to coincide with available

resources, and delay some components until additional resources are available.

- **Goals of the needs assessment.**
  The goals of the assessment should be reviewed in light of the coalition's goals. It is important to decide how extensive your assessment will be — in other words, how wide a net to cast. Assembling a picture of all youth problems and youth services in a community is a major task. Adolescent pregnancy (the problem both as it exists and as it is perceived), along with existing services, needs to be placed in the context of other youth issues. Trying to achieve equal depth on all youth issues, however, will exhaust your resources unless your coalition has explicitly concluded that this is needed, will be useful, and is "doable."

Your information-gathering activities may vary in complexity and comprehensiveness depending upon your purposes and resources. However extensive your data collection methods, it is important to know ahead of time how the information will be analyzed and presented. This helps insure that you collect pertinent and accessible information.

A Road Map

The needs assessment will help you create a clear profile of the adolescent pregnancy problem and its indicators in your community. The demographic data you collect and the profile of available service options for teenagers will help you put together a current picture. The opinions of key community participants, including teenagers, parents, adults, professionals, and other community leaders, will help create guide-posts and a sense of direction for community efforts. The following sections are intended to address the kinds of questions that need to be answered to develop a comprehensive community-wide plan.

Examples of Needs Assessment Questions

The purpose of a community-wide assessment is to begin answering a set of questions that your agency or coalition believes are important. The information gleaned from this process becomes the core for program planning. This information is not static. It changes often, sometimes overnight. An ongoing monitoring of information ensures that the data utilized for program planning are appropriate. A source of current data is also important when fine-tuning programs that are already in place.

A variety of questions may be asked during an effective needs assessment. Many of the guiding questions in this section and at the end of this chapter (Appendix 5-2) have been adapted from the Children's Defense Fund Adolescent Pregnancy Childwatch Manual (1987). They can help you determine what information to obtain for your community's needs assessment. You will probably not find answers to all these questions, but the framework should help you decide the questions most relevant to your specific community.

Demographic Profile

You should begin by developing a general demographic profile of the community and then a specific profile on the incidence of adolescent pregnancy and births. Of all the information you seek in your assessment, you will find that demographic data (e.g. age, race, incidence of births) are the easiest to collect. However, demographic data will only partly illuminate the picture of adolescent pregnancy in the community. You should also gather data on other important factors that contribute to the social and economic profile of your community (such as the incidence of poverty, the numbers of adolescents and young children being raised by single parents, the amount of public housing available, and the health status of adolescents). This information must be added to the demographic statistics. Your overall goal is to identify the nature of the problem in the community, and the groups that are in the greatest need of services. Chart 5-1 summarizes examples of questions that will help you gather information on the extent of the problem in your community.

Chart 5-1

Developing a Demographic Profile of Adolescent Pregnancy in the Community

- Number of total live births, by race.

- Number of male and female adolescents ages 12-19 living in the community, by age and race.

- Number of adolescent abortions, by race and age.

- Number of births to adolescents, by race and age. If at all possible, seek information for specific ages, such as for 13, 14, 15, 16, 17, etc., rather than an aggregate of data such as ages 15-19.

- Number of first and subsequent births (parity, or birth order) to adolescents by race and age.

- Number of births to unmarried adolescents, by race and age.

- Number of adolescents who received prenatal care, by race, and when prenatal care began.

- Number of babies with low birthweight (less than 2500 grams or 5 1/2 pounds) born to adolescent mothers, by race and by age of mother.

Community Resources

The needs assessment process should help you determine which agency or combination of agencies would be most appropriate to develop or implement a set of strategies. It should also allow you to identify gaps in services and resources. You may find that even existing agencies require additional resources to expand their capacity to respond to the problems you have identified.

Examples of questions that will help you identify the extent of community resources and their utilization are listed below:

- How many adolescents receive family planning services in the community?

- How many adolescents receive health and mental health care (by major provider of care) in the community?

- Have any private organizations or advocacy groups taken an active role in addressing the issue of adolescent pregnancy and pregnancy prevention? Specify the groups, their activities, their target population, and the outcomes of their efforts.

- To what extent are current efforts devoted to the treatment and amelioration of the problem, rather than placing a priority on primary prevention?

- Are there any public and/or private programs relating to pregnancy prevention operating within or associated with the schools? Within other community settings?

- Are there any public and/or private programs for employment training and placement of students who have dropped out or who are on the verge of dropping out of school? Specify who the providers are; the type of training and jobs that are available; outreach and access to the program; numbers of participants by age, sex, and race/ethnicity; number of adolescents on waiting lists; number of adolescents who have been successfully placed in jobs; and funding sources of programs. Is there any coordination with school programs?

- What are the specific community resources that are currently allocated to the issue (e.g. public and private funding including federal, state, local and foundation support, in kind support, number of volunteers, etc.)?

Adolescents at Risk of Pregnancy and Other Risk Behaviors

Your needs assessment should include a series of questions about the life of adolescents in your community. The goal is to create a profile of at-risk adolescents. While not all students who drop out of school face an early unintended pregnancy, recent studies indicate that a number of factors appear to be both the antecedents and the consequences of adolescent pregnancy. Data on such factors as educational and employment status of young people are telling indicators of unmet need. The following questions will also help identify youths who are at risk:

- What percentage of students is behind for age in their grade placement, by class and school?

- What percentage of students is experiencing school failure, by class and school?

- What percentage of students is dropping out of school, by age and school?

- What is the employment rate for young people in the community, both for part-time and full-time work?

- What are the labor participation rates for young people in the community?

- How many young people are enrolled in special job training programs?

- How many youths live in out-of-home placements, including foster care?

- How many are held in police detention at least once a year?

- What are the annual numbers of arrests for substance abuse and for drunken driving?

- How many emergency room visits were made by adolescents, and what were the primary reasons for their visits?

- How many were arrested for juvenile delinquency?

- What is the incidence of runaway youths?

- How many adolescents are enrolled in substance abuse treatment programs, both hospital and out-patient services?

General Information Questions to Ask All Providers

Opinions and attitudes of community representatives are useful for understanding the problems you are investigating. Both objective data and opinions help to create a multidimensional, and thus more accurate, picture of needs. Interviews should be conducted with professionals who work directly with adolescents, professionals in health and social service programs, leaders in local and county governments, business and industrial leaders, representatives of political parties, minority representatives, college faculty in departments relating to adolescents, leaders in civic clubs, media representatives, members of voluntary youth-serving organizations, parents, and adolescents (Children's Defense Fund, Childwatch Manual, 1987). Depending on whether you conduct a written survey or personal interviews, you may select an open-ended or closed-ended questionnaire format (see Chapter 8 on Evaluation for suggestions on questionnaire format). Open-ended interviews will be particularly useful if you are doing an exploratory study, while closed-ended questions can be more easily analyzed. The following questions (posed as open-ended ones here) are examples that you may wish to use in order to assess perceptions of community leaders.

- What do you believe are the most critical problems or the greatest unmet needs facing young people in the community? What do you believe are their underlying causes? On a local level, what do you view as the biggest obstacle to solving each of these problems?

- What do you believe should be done to resolve these barriers and how are you involved in the solution to these problems?

- How concerned do you think the residents of the area are about each of these problems? Who do you feel are the most knowledgeable people in each of these problem areas?

- What local adolescent pregnancy prevention programs do you feel have been successful in your community? Why are they successful? What are your conclusions based on?

The following sections will help guide those conducting the needs assessment process in identifying data collection approaches and sources of information.

Sources of Needs Assessment Data

Data for your needs assessment can come from a variety of sources. In fact, using multiple sources of information will likely increase the accuracy of your assessment. The sources discussed below vary in the formality of data collection and in the depth of the picture they offer. Used in combination, however, they can help you create a comprehensive perspective of your target population. When your sources begin to converge and substantiate each other, you can be more confident that the data are complete. Continue to work with an advisory group and with representatives of the groups you survey, whether informal or formal, to help verify whether the information you are collecting is truly reflective of the problems as these groups perceive them.

In a relatively uncharted area such as pregnancy prevention, you will need to collect data that document the current incidence of adolescent births in the community, as well as the impact of the problem on the next generation of adolescents if community-wide strategies are not implemented. It is also crucial to collect state and federal data on the incidence of adolescent pregnancy in order to be able to compare your own community against a broader profile. This information will also help you assess to what degree your community is being affected by this important issue.

Public Documents and Statistics

These data sources are most useful in obtaining a demographic, economic, social, and reproductive profile of the community.

Census data, available in libraries or for purchase directly from the Census Bureau, provide the incidence of poverty, number of single heads of household, unemployment rates, education completion, and the age, gender, language, and ethnic distribution of each county. Some of these measures can help establish the need for a program in your community. Look in the "General Social and Economic Characteristics" volume for your state in the *Census of Population* for this information.

A drawback to using census data is the time lag between collection of the data and their availability to the public; major census data are collected only every ten years. However, the Census Bureau conducts regional studies in other time sequences. Data by smaller areas — for example, by zip code and census tract — are often available through local planning agencies, councils, and commissions. Other resources include departments of vital statistics within health departments, urban affairs departments, public service institutes, programs at universities, and central libraries.

Vital statistics include county birth and death certificates, which can be used to document the birth rate for a target group, incidence of low birthweight, mortality, and morbidity. Some states also include information on when prenatal care was begun. Data from hospitals and county health departments can supplement this data and keep you up to date on changes the community may be undergoing.

Other resources are yearly reports prepared by cities or counties that describe their problems, needs, priorities, programs, resources, and plans. These reports will provide insights into funding priorities and will also enable you to target your activities to unmet needs, and to avoid duplication or conflicts with programs already planned. They may also include budgetary information, such as early warning of budgetary cuts that may place restrictions on access to family planning services for adolescents. State agencies may have other reports and studies that will be of interest to your group.

The school district office or individual schools may be a source of such information as school dropout rates, truancy, suspensions, school nurse reports, and probation status of students. This information will help you identify adolescents at high risk of pregnancy. Contact the local principal or superintendent's office, or the state department of education. The information you need may not always exist in formal documents. When formal data do not exist, it may be helpful to conduct informal interviews with school personnel, including principals, teachers, counselors, psychologists, social workers, and nurses, as well as with parents and students. Special and alternative schools, and private and parochial schools should be included in addition to regular public schools. Personal contact (e.g., phone, visit) with school leaders is usually the most effective way to obtain information.

The Chamber of Commerce, as well as local marketing researchers and pollsters, may possess useful demographic data. Their reports, though not specifically health related, may include profiles of the growth of new populations and economic shifts in employment that will provide insights into your community. If money is available, community groups can pay to have questions added to ongoing public opinion surveys; this can be a cost-effective way to gather limited data from a large and representative population.

Other Sources of
Community
Information

Many of the following agencies may have collected community information that will be helpful in developing a profile:

- Local, county, state, and federal departments of health, education, probation, and social services.

- Representatives of local, state, and federal government agencies that are responsible for programs and activities in the areas of human resources, social services, child welfare, and public income supports. Programs include Aid to Families with Dependent Children, social block grants, foster care, departments of social services or public welfare, the Human Resources Administration, and the Children's Bureau. In addition, other agencies that perform services for children and their families exist in county and city governments. Along with interviews, be sure to collect literature, studies, and evaluations of programs relating to adolescent pregnancy prevention.

- City and regional planning agencies.

- Adolescent health programs.

- Family planning agencies.

- Medical societies, including the American Association of Pediatrics and the American Association of Obstetricians and Gynecologists.

- Community action agencies, health and welfare councils.

- Community organizations (PTA, League of Women Voters, American Association of University Women, etc.).

- Community and state colleges and universities.

- Major employers.

- Umbrella organizations such as United Way.

- Adolescent pregnancy coalitions, networks, or programs operating in your community, county, or state. Other national organizations or advocacy organizations, such as the Children's Defense Fund, Center for Population Options, March of Dimes, National Organization on Adolescent Pregnancy and Parenting, etc., may be knowledgeable of individuals within your area who are either involved in developing coalitions or who are interested in youth issues. It is important to identify potential organizations and/or individuals with whom you can create stronger alliances and coalitions.

- Youth or child advocacy organizations.

- Youth-serving agencies, e.g. Boys Clubs/Girls Clubs, Boy Scouts/Girl Scouts, Camp Fire Girls, YWCAs and YMCAs, etc.

- Civil rights and minority social service organizations, such as the Urban League, Delta Sigma Theta, La Raza, League of United Latin American Citizens, etc.

- Religious organizations, including Catholic Social Services, Salvation Army, Lutheran Social Services, Council of Jewish Women, as well as churches and synagogues.

- Recreational programs.

- Libraries.

- Women's organizations, such as the Junior League and Zeta Phi Beta sorority.

Legislative resources. Visit your local state senate or assembly representatives and ask for their ideas regarding adolescent pregnancy prevention. Then ask to be introduced to the chairperson of the legislative subcommittee on health, maternal and child health, and/or youth. Ask the chairperson whom he or she seeks out for input on adolescent pregnancy related matters, and whom he or she considers to be the most knowledgeable in the area of youth. In addition, contact your local mayor and members of the city council to ask for their advice.

Journal and newspaper articles. Journal and newspaper articles (especially local ones), reference manuals, and clearinghouse information can provide in-depth descriptions of the problem and offer potential solutions, although some may not be specific to your community.

Surveys and interviews. Written surveys and interviews with adolescents, health providers, and teachers will enable you to obtain the opinion of many individuals on a given topic. School-wide needs assessment questionnaires have been used successfully to document the need for school-based and school-linked services. These methods of data collection allow you to involve potential consumers in the needs assessment process and also to educate the community about available and needed services. Interviews, although they reach fewer people than written surveys, usually elicit in-depth information.

When designing the survey or interview questionnaire, care must be taken to allow for a wide variance of opinion on the problem and potential solutions. You must also take care to survey a representative sample of the population. If other needs assessments are currently underway, you may be able to work collaboratively, or ask that your survey questions be included. In exchange, you can help in tallying information.

Observation visits. Statistics, reports, and secondhand interpretations can never replace personal observations. There is no better way to obtain a full understanding of the scope of a problem, such as poverty, inadequate education, or unemployment, than to visit the communities involved. Direct observation of clinics and health centers, schools, community recreation settings, and other sites is an important part of the needs assessment process.

Planning observation visits is similar to conducting interviews. For formal agency visits, it may be helpful to conduct interviews or obtain background information, such as agency reports and brochures before the visit. Be sure the number of observers does not impose on the agency; if multiple observers wish to conduct visits, it is much better to send several small groups than one large one. After the visit, observers should share their impressions and one member should prepare a report for future reference.

Focus groups are exploratory group sessions that afford insights into a target population's perceptions and beliefs. Focus groups can be held selectively with adolescents, professionals, and community leaders, and may be useful both in the needs assessment process and in the early stages of program development. Sessions can be conducted with a group of about eight to ten participants. Using a discussion outline, a moderator keeps the session on track, allowing participants to talk freely about the topic of interest. Ideally, focus group participants do not know other members of the group, as this may inhibit expression. Some small incentive to participate in a session (gift, money, etc.) may be useful in recruiting.

As with respondent groups for written surveys, the choice of focus group participants should reflect the intended target group. Subgroups (by ethnicity, gender, age) within your target population should be represented. However, when discussing a sensitive subject such as sexuality, you may want to segregate groups by age and sex to encourage full participation. For example, teenage girls may be less open talking about contraception if parents or teenage boys are in the group. A discussion about communication, on the other hand, may be enhanced by the interplay within a mixed group.

While there is no rule as to how many focus groups are necessary, four should be enough if the groups are representative of the target population. Each session should be recorded for later review and interpretation. Look for trends and patterns in participants' beliefs and opinions when analyzing results.

Developing Your Information Matrix

Before you start to collect data, it is helpful to develop a matrix, or information chart. As you fill in the matrix you can get a sense of how many sources will be necessary and what information should be gathered from each. In addition, use of the matrix will help avoid unnecessary duplication of effort, and ensure that the data gathering efforts have been thorough. Once you know which questions need to be asked, write them on the left part of the matrix. At the top of the page, in column headings, write down the best source of data for each question and the best ways to collect the information. (See Worksheet 5-3 at the end of this chapter. Worksheets 5-1 and 5-2 also show how to construct charts to summarize data collected from interviews and surveys.)

Preparing the Questions

Needs assessment questions should be tailored to your particular community to help uncover underlying gaps in services and potential resources. As you review the list of questions in the Needs Assessment Questionnaire Guide in Appendix 5-2, consider having a set of core questions to be asked of every participant, and a separate set of questions to delve into the specifics of the organizations under review. The questions presented in this chapter are worded in such a manner that they can be asked of a variety of umbrella organizations which may or may not have specific program details. In interviews with service-oriented organizations and agencies, word your questions to fit the functions of the specific organizations. For example, rather than asking a YMCA representative about all the activities in your community, ask first about specific activities *they* provide to adolescents and then whether they are aware of other organizations that serve their target populations. Especially in the area of adolescent pregnancy prevention, questions should be focused on both primary prevention efforts, such as sexuality education and the availability and accessibility of contraceptive services, and on efforts that may be considered peripheral to the issue of adolescent pregnancy prevention, such as the availability of recreational activities, school tutoring, and other after school programs. Both kinds of efforts are important aspects of a community-wide adolescent pregnancy prevention strategy.

It is also important to distinguish among: 1) adolescents who are not pregnant or parenting; 2) pregnant adolescents and their partners; and 3) parenting adolescents. While you may wish to document what your community provides for the latter two categories, the overall focus of this needs assessment is on primary prevention.

Inevitably, some information will be difficult to obtain. Be persistent and clear about your goals. Many organizations or agencies, such as schools, do not keep good records, thus the information is not readily available. You may find that establishing a mechanism for data collection will be a major recommendation that emerges from your study.

Many communities and states have a task force on children, adolescents, or adolescent pregnancy. This task force may be collecting information that can be included in your needs assessment. Once these departments and programs are identified, interview the agency directors to assess policies and programs that have been established. For purposes of the needs assessment, finding that no specific program or effort is in place may be as valuable as learning about specific programs. The purpose is to identify gaps in programatic efforts and to identify potential ways to eliminate those gaps.

Developing a Workplan

You and your committee have now established the set of questions you will explore, the data that you want to collect, and the agencies you will contact. Implementation of your planned needs assessment will most likely require a number of individuals to conduct the data-gathering phase. You will also need to develop a detailed timeline for completing all your tasks. Finally, you must establish how to analyze and report your findings. As you determine which data your needs assessment will utilize, it is important to differentiate between the data collected from interviews and that from written sources of information, such as school reports and county data. These data collection sources call into play different types of skills and require different time commitments. Be sure that your data collection efforts are conducted in a careful and methodical manner, and conscientiously document the sources of your data.

Training Interviewers

Whether you use staff or volunteers to collect the needs assessment data, it is important that adequate training be provided, particularly for those involved in conducting surveys and interviews. Interviewers must thoroughly understand the questions that they are going to ask, or they will be unable to clarify them for the person being interviewed. Interviewer training should include an explanation of the survey's purpose, what is meant by each question, and why the information is needed, as well as opportunities to role-play and practice interviewing. Consider using interviewing teams of two, with one person asking the questions and the other recording the answers. This can save time, and assure more consistent information recording. It may also be useful to have two impressions of the interview.

The training should also include practical suggestions for gaining entry into organizations. It is important to obtain administrative support for your efforts, especially if the interview team is interviewing direct-service providers. You can either call or write to set up an appointment. Allow enough time to collect data in a thorough manner, but keep to a reasonable time limit since you will often be talking to busy people with many competing demands on their time.

The interviewers may find that they have to be persistent in setting up appointments. Interviewers need to establish the credibility of the needs assessment effort. They can explain why the interview is important in the data collection phase of the project. It may also help to have available an information sheet describing your organization or coalition, the purpose for the survey, and the anticipated use of the results. Many interviewees will want to have access to the data you are collecting. This is also a good opportunity to assess the potential for collaboration during the planning and implementation phases of the project.

*Deciding Whom
to Interview*

You will want to interview a variety of agency and community representatives during
your needs assessment process. Be sure to include individuals from agencies that
serve a range of geographic and income areas in the community. Given the large
number of organizations in many communities, it is important that the team conducting the needs assessment give careful thought to the question of which agencies will
be contacted.

Planning and advocacy organizations are probably the best preliminary sources to
approach because they usually possess a wide view of what is happening in the
community. For example, the first interviews may take place with representatives from
such community-based umbrella organizations as the United Way, an adolescent
pregnancy coalition, and a youth or child advocacy organization. These agencies
should be able to direct you to a variety of other organizations and people in the
community who are knowledgeable about adolescent pregnancy issues (see
Children's Defense Fund: *Childwatch Manual*, 1987).

Ideally, a population-based study (conducting door-to-door interviews of randomly-
selected households) will provide the most insightful picture of a community's needs.
However, in reality we are often limited to gathering data drawn from individuals who
have come into contact with the system of agencies or providers of care. That is why
an advisory board or coalition that allows for valuable feedback from potential clients
and community representatives is essential to verify the validity of the community
profile you are assembling.

To compensate those you interviewed for their cooperation, and also raise the level of
awareness within the community, write a short report on how and why the survey was
conducted, and send this report, with a copy of the questions and the results, to all
survey participants.

*Protection of
Human Rights*

It is the responsibility of those conducting the needs assessment to prevent anyone
from using the information provided by the respondents to harm them in any way. For
that reason it is highly important to guard the confidentiality of information provided
by survey participants.

If you are collecting surveys from community residents, completed questionnaires
should be identified by code numbers instead of names. Potential participants should
be assured that their names will not be on the questionnaire, that they have the right
to refuse to participate, and that they may refuse to answer any particular question.
You may wish to hand the participant a list of these assurances, along with the name
and phone number of the person in charge of the project for contact at a later date if
participants have any questions. You can leave space at the bottom of this list for
respondents to sign after they have read their rights, formally agreeing to participate
in the interview. One copy of this consent form should be left with the participant and
one copy should be kept in your files.

Building Trust

It is important to establish trust within your community during the needs assessment process. Be sure that you explain to people why you (and the community) need the information that you are collecting, how the data will be used, and what potential benefits to the community may accrue as a result of the assessment. Communities may fear a needs assessment process because of concerns about how the information will be used, and about your motivation for collecting it. Members of the coalition will be particularly useful in helping you identify the best way to collect information without alienating the community. It is also important to identify the interviewer who will be most effective at eliciting information from each potential information source. Under certain circumstances it may be wise to ensure that at least one member of the interview team is a member of the target community. Interviews should also document requests made by those who are interviewed about participating in the project, or helping to determine how the information will be used.

The Needs Assessment Report

Collecting information without careful notes is a waste of time and will not contribute toward developing an effective report. The best approach is to record the collected information immediately following each step of the needs assessment. Be sure to include the date, pertinent information about persons talked to, their responses to questions, and a summary of your impressions. Intermediate reports should be shared with others conducting the assessment so they can utilize the information to probe further as they conduct their interviews. Follow up with any action items resulting from the interview, such as setting up additional interviews with individuals identified during the interview, gathering a report that was referred to during the interview, etc.

Analyze answers from different people by placing all answers to each individual question side by side to assess consistencies and inconsistencies. The needs assessment report should include a short summary, methods (what did you do, how did you do it, who did it, and when it was done), and findings (responses to questions, observations, problems discovered, resources available, potential obstacles, and possible ways to overcome them).

Using Needs Assessment Data to Increase Interagency Cooperation

Since the agency resources available to conduct a community assessment are generally limited, you may want to share the community-based needs assessment data with specific human services agencies serving the same geographic area. The information you gather can also be used to identify areas in which cooperative sharing of available services from different agencies can effectively meet a community need, while avoiding the creation of duplicate services. Data can be used by agency personnel, boards of directors, and funding sources to analyze services in the community. And data can also be used to demonstrate the need and the means for developing specific services in a given catchment area where they may not be presently available. The data effectively lend themselves to the idea of cooperative planning and service delivery, a concept too frequently overlooked in the field of human services. Chapter 6 offers additional suggestions for utilizing the data you have collected.

*Preparing and
Disseminating Your
Report*

As you prepare the needs assessment report, distribute a draft form to representatives of coalition or core agencies comprising the planning group for their comments and critique. Once the changes and corrections have been made, a final report can be prepared and distributed.

The needs assessment report may continue to serve as an internal working document and be used for grant-writing purposes. Once specific strategies are adopted, it becomes a baseline document against which program development and implementation can be measured. It can also be used as a public document, widely disseminated to both public and private agencies as an indication of unmet needs in the community, and as a starting place for further coalition building (Children's Defense Fund, *Childwatch Manual*, 1987). Needs assessments are also important for process-monitoring and for maintaining a pulse on changing community needs, perceptions, and priorities. While it may not be an objective for your coalition to target all the identified service gaps uncovered, it may be beneficial to other groups to have your findings so that they can advocate for changes and new programs in related areas. For example, while it may not be feasible for your coalition to start a job training program, other community agencies may identify a potential source of funding for developing such a program. While these efforts may not be related specifically to adolescent pregnancy, they will contribute to changing the overall climate for youth in the community.

Brief documents that visually summarize your findings become powerful tools. For example, maps can be used to illustrate areas with high rates of adolescent births, low-birthweight babies, school dropouts, youth unemployment, etc. They can also be used to show potential locations of programs and the projected impact of these programs on the target population. Other visual tools to summarize data may include bar and line graphs. Bar graphs are often used for showing comparisons or contrasts; for example, local statistics in relation to state and national figures. They can also show how teenage births are broken down by age of the mother, or by the numbers of young people enrolled in a variety of community programs. Line graphs may be used to illustrate change over a number of years, or the effects of one variable on another, such as the number of adolescent births over the past ten years in a community, or the impact of different kinds of educational program interventions on school dropout rates. Information from interviews and observations may be harder to present in graphics, but can be presented in summaries and in original quotations. Salient quotes are often helpful in supporting data, tying the human experience to the numbers you have collected.

You may wish to make a summary report of your findings available for wide distribution to policy makers such as legislators, program planners, program managers, and others, including funding sources. The summary report should include a clear statement of the goals of the project, a description of the lead agency and other sponsoring agencies and organizations, and an explanation of how data were collected. The report should also include a summary of the community's pregnancy prevention programs and activities, including some details as to what services they provide and whom they serve. Major issues and unmet needs should be identified, and recommendations and follow-up activities should be noted. Based on the data that have been collected throughout the needs assessment process, you may draw conclusions as to the extent of the problem in your community, particularly as compared to the standards the community wants to establish in the area of adolescent pregnancy prevention (see Chapter 4 for a good example of community standards in adolescent pregnancy prevention). The needs assessment process will have helped sort out who is most affected by the problem, what is currently being done to alleviate or solve it, and what factors are contributing to a worsening of the problem. All this combined information must be blended into a "problem statement," which clearly spells out a message leading to action. The report or a summary should be provided to all participating agencies and other individuals who have indicated throughout the needs assessment process that they are interested in participating in follow-up activities. In addition to the complete report, which at 50-100 pages may be too long for most people to read, develop a fact sheet such as the one on page 135, outlining the most important findings in language that is easily understood. Try to place these fact sheets where they are accessible to all community members, such as in libraries and community health clinics. You may consider sending them to parents of junior-high and high-school-age children. When you make presentations to community groups, hand them out for people to take home to share with friends and neighbors.

Next Steps

As a coordinated community-wide adolescent pregnancy prevention plan emerges to address the identified needs, providers will confront the fiscal realities of implementing new programs. In view of such fiscal realities as finite funding, program planning that is based on (and statistically supported by) accurate needs assessment data becomes even more essential; data are available to demonstrate the need and to support the suggested programming strategy for reducing the identified problems. While available funding may be fixed, priorities established through the needs assessment process may help set the direction for reallocation of funding.

The program planning process uses the information obtained in the needs assessment to create focused goals and objectives for a program that responds to the identified needs. A comprehensive plan will also include the establishment of standards for the program's outcome, a timetable, methods of integrating the program with existing programs, and establishment of a referral system outlining how individuals will enter and exit from the program. The needs assessment process will yield a massive amount of information, which must be categorized both to determine a program focus and to set priorities for that focus.

Overall, the direction should be toward developing comprehensive care for youth, coordination of services, and avoidance of duplication.

Factsheet

Anytown Teen Life Coalition:
Adolescent Pregnancy Fact Sheet

Background: In March of this year a coalition of agencies concerned with the rate of teen pregnancies in Anytown conducted an assessment of the problem. A summary of the results is outlined below.

- Last year in Anytown, 593 teenagers between the ages of 15 and 19 had babies. That means **1 out of every 20 girls in this age group gave birth.**

- **70% of the girls who had a child dropped out of school,** thus limiting their chances of obtaining a fulfilling job with which they can support a family. Nationally, only 46% of female teens who drop out of school return to obtain their diploma or go back for their GED.

- In a survey of the local high schools, **60% of students reported being sexually active.**

- Of those teens who reported being sexually active, only **35% had used contraception** the last time they had intercourse.

- In a survey of parents, community members, and agencies working with adolescents, **teen pregnancy was among the top three concerns** they had for teenagers. Drug use and school drop-out were the other two top concerns.

In response to these findings, the Anytown Teen Life Coalition will be working on strategies to support our community's teenagers. If you would like to work with us in designing and implementing programs, or if you would like to receive a more detailed report, please call us at (telephone).

Summary

The needs assessment chronicles both need and unmet need. It should provide a profile of the adolescent pregnancy problem and its indicators in the community. In order to tailor the coalition's plan to the particular community, it is vital that the group document local circumstances in relation to teenage childbearing — to come to know its own adolescents and all existing organizations that serve them. Decisions that must be made prior to conducting the study include: (1) a determination of the goals of the study, (2) a clear definition of the target community, (3) decisions about what kind of standards the community should achieve, (4) a consensus about the scope of the assessment, and (5) the identification of resources that will be useful in conducting the study.

The assessment team should begin by constructing a demographic profile, including a clear identification of adolescents at risk of pregnancy as well as other risk behaviors. A variety of sources both public and private have been suggested here as possible resources for community projects. A plan or matrix developed beforehand will help to ensure thoroughness in data gathering and avoiding duplication. The information gathered must eventually be synthesized into a needs assessment report, which will be an important tool for the coalition's planning and decision-making process. It also will serve as a valuable tool in gaining credibility and support from community groups and funding sources. The next chapter provides an outline for translating the needs assessment findings into a comprehensive strategy.

Appendix 5-1

A Guide for Calculating a Community's Birthrate

*T*his guide will assist you in calculating the birthrate for a community. In the following case the community is defined as a total county, but the same calculations can also be made for smaller geographic areas if you have access to the requisite data.

Birthrates by age of mother can be obtained from most county departments of health in your state. Ask for age-specific birth rates by age of mother, either by zip code or by census tract. This detailed information provides a fertility picture for your community. For example, it can help you assess what proportion of 16-year-olds are having children in each part of your community each year.

If a table of birth rates is not available, obtain the table of live births by age of mother for the target communities. This table will not give rates of births (per 1,000 women), but only absolute numbers of births per age group. In order to calculate the birthrate (live births per 1,000 women) for your community, divide the number of live births by the number of women in the age group you are interested in reaching.

$$\text{Birthrate} = \frac{\text{Number of live births to women in specified group}}{\text{Number of women in specified group}} \times 1,000$$

To obtain the table of population projections listed by individual ages (14, 15, 16, 17, etc.) and by gender (male and female) for a specified year for your county, call the population research unit within your state.

Example

To calculate the 1988 birth rate for a certain county for women ages 15-19:

Step 1: Sum the number of live births for 15, 16, 17, 18, and 19-year-olds. For example:

$$105 + 214 + 314 + 477 + 639 = 1749$$

Step 2: Look up the estimated female population of 15- to 19-year-olds for 1988. For example:

$$15\text{- to } 19\text{-year-old women} = 46,600$$

Step 3: Divide the number obtained in Step 1 by that obtained in Step 2 and multiply by 1000. This is the birthrate for 15- to 19-year-old women for the county.

$$(1749 \div 46,600) \times 1,000 = 37.5$$

Appendix 5-2

Needs Assessment Data Collection Guide

Demographic and Socioeconomic Profile

*T*o establish trends in your community, it is best to seek data for the years beginning 20 years ago and continuing in 5-year increments (i.e., 1975, 1980, 1985, 1990, or the most recently available years). This will help reveal whether there are changes or new trends of which your community should be made aware.

General Demographic and Socioeconomic Profile

- What is the total population of your state, county, and/or city for each race/ethnicity, age, and sex?

- What are the numbers of adolescents living in your target community, by race/ethnicity, age (e.g. 10-14, 15-17, and 18-19-year-olds), and sex?

  In some sites, you may wish to collect individual year data to compare the potential pool of adolescents at risk of pregnancy with the incidence of adolescent births by year.

- What are the population projections into the year 2000? Is there a trend toward increasing or decreasing numbers of adolescents residing in the community? What is the overall proportion of adolescents to the population in general?

- How many adolescents and young adults (20-24) are employed?

- What is the average income level for the community? What is the incidence of poverty in the community? What percentage of adolescents and pre-adolescents are living in poverty? What proportion of adolescents live in households headed by only one parent?

- What is the extent of subsidized housing in your community? What is the degree of homelessness for young people? (Note: Estimates for this number are acceptable as homelessness is difficult to document; a range of numbers provided should be shown as part of your summary).

Adolescent Fertility

- What is the total number of live births, by race?

- What is the number of births to adolescents, by race and age? (If at all possible, obtain data for specific ages, e.g. 15-, 16-, 17-year-olds, etc., rather than aggregate totals, e.g. ages 15-19).

- What is the number of first and subsequent births (parity or birth order) to adolescents, by race and by age?

- What is the number of births to unmarried adolescents, by race and by age?

- What is the number of adolescents who receive prenatal care, by race, and when did prenatal care begin?

- What is the number of babies with low birthweight (less than 2500 grams or 5 1/2 pounds) born to adolescent mothers, by race and by age of mother?

- What is the number of abortions performed on adolescents, by race and by age. (Note: Not all communities collect this information, and you may have to rely on the estimates developed for various states by the Alan Guttmacher Institute and the Centers for Disease Control).

Health and Other Factors

- What are the rates of reportable sexually transmitted diseases among youths, by age and gender?

- What number of adolescents receive family planning services in the community?

- What number of adolescents receive health and mental health care (by major provider of care) in the community?

- What is the known incidence of uninsurance or under-insurance for the community in general and for adolescents in particular?

- Are there any special nutrition and/or medical services for adolescents provided in the schools, community health clinics, or at other sites?

- Does receipt of any public financial assistance automatically entitle adolescents to any health services? For example, if an adolescent receives AFDC, is he/she also eligible for Medicaid?

• What number of adolescents receive health screening by Early Periodic Screening and Detection and Treatment services (EPSDT)? How many of these adolescents are referred for additional medical services?

School-related Issues

• What is the incidence of school dropout, by age, sex, and race/ethnicity? What is the number of adolescents who drop out in the transition between junior high and high school? What are the primary reasons for dropping out of school? How is dropout information collected for the school district, and what constitutes a definition of "dropout"? What are the dropout trends in the school district over the past five years?

• How many students are absent more than 25% of the semester, by major cause of absenteeism, age, race, and sex?

• What percentage of students are held back? What percentage of students have low test scores?

• What schools have a high academic failure rate in the community?

• If the school district offers dropout prevention programs, including alternative high schools, how many students are currently enrolled in these programs? How many students are on waiting lists for these programs?

• How many pregnant school dropouts are known to return to school after they deliver their babies? How many infant or toddler childcare slots are available to these students?

Other Youth Populations

• What is the rate of employment for young people in the community?

• How many young people are enrolled in special job training programs?

• How many young people are in out-of-home placements, including foster care?

• How many young people are held in detention at least once a year?

• What are the numbers of arrests of young people for substance abuse and for drunken driving?

• What is the number of juvenile delinquency arrests?

• What is the incidence of adolescent runaway youths?

• What are the numbers of adolescents enrolled in substance abuse treatment programs, both hospital and out-patient services?

**Available
Community
Resources**

- What kinds of activities are community agencies, such as the YMCA, Girls Clubs and Boys Clubs, Big Brother/Big Sister, community centers, Urban League, church groups, etc., providing to adolescents and preadolescents in the following areas:

  a) Development of self-concept and self-esteem building

  b) Life planning and counseling

  c) Family life education, including communication skills, interpersonal relationships, contraceptive information, sources for contraceptive care, etc.

  d) Job training

  e) Mentoring programs

  f) Recreational activities

  g) Other (please describe)

  For each of these areas, it is important to gather program information that includes:

  - Age, race, and sex of participants

  - Types of specific activities

  - Providers of care

  - Access to services, including eligibility requirements, hours, location, transportation, parental consent, cost of participating in the activity for adolescents and their families

  - Outreach efforts, including community recruitment, advertisement, and other techniques used to encourage participation

  - Funding sources utilized, including public and private funding.

- Which of the above activities are specifically targeted to males? Please describe these programs in detail, particularly the outreach efforts that have been adopted.

- Do parents of teenagers participate in any of the above youth-oriented activities?

- Are there programs or activities (e.g., workshops, seminars, courses, etc.) on adolescent pregnancy prevention or life planning that are geared to parents of teenagers or preadolescents? If there are, specify program activity, duration of activity, providers, numbers of participants, race/ethnicity and sex of participants, access, outreach, and funding source.

- What family counseling or crisis service centers for families in stress are available in your community? Are there any centers targeted specifically to adolescents and their families (include fee structure and accessibility requirements)?

School System Resources

Family Life Education

- What school-sponsored courses and activities (e.g. assemblies, class projects, etc.) address family life education and pregnancy prevention? (Include activities on the elementary, junior, and senior high levels.) Specifically, which of the following topics are covered?

    a) Sex education (e.g., family life, health, sexuality)

    b) Family planning

    c) Child care

    d) Child development

    e) Parenting/marriage

    f) Nutrition education

- For each of the above, please specify the type of activity, courses, grade level, number of participants by age and sex, types of providers involved, access and outreach, frequency and duration of activity(s), and funding sources used, within both the school budget and the non-school budget.

- What school personnel have been assigned responsibility for these activities (include the administrative position and the required training)?

- How extensive is the family life education program in terms of what specific topics are included (for example, self-esteem, communication skills, life planning, birth control methods, where services can be received in the community) etc.?

- When is family life education introduced in the curriculum and what is its length? For example, are educational efforts semester-long classes or "one-shot" lectures by outside agency educators? What specific age groups are targeted for these efforts?

- Who provides this information in the schools — is it part of the established curriculum taught by the teachers, or do teachers rely on other school staff (e.g., school nurse) or outside agencies to provide the information, or are both resources utilized? Do teachers receive special training in family life education? If so, for how long and where is this training received?

- Are there any other kinds of sex education and family life education programs, such as information hot lines, available in the community?

- Are educational efforts coordinated? For example, is there a centralized speaker's bureau composed of all the community's health educators?

- What community agencies teach in the classroom? In what other sites do these agencies provide their information?

- How many parents withhold their permission, thus preventing their children from attending these educational sessions?

- Have past family life education efforts been effective with this target population or other at-risk populations in the community? What results have been documented in your evaluations? What techniques have been the most effective in reaching your audience?

Life Options

- List the school system's offerings, if any, under the following headings:

  a) Career planning counseling and courses

  b) Compensatory education programs, such as tutoring, remedial, or other special courses

  c) Vocational education

  d) Job placement

  e) Community service placements

  f) Other special efforts designed to keep adolescents in school

- What activities do community-based organizations, such as Girls and Boys Clubs, sponsor that aim at broadening the life options of their clients? For example, do they offer introductions to different careers, learning about community resources, experiences attending cultural events, etc.?

- Are there any joint activities between schools and community-based agencies, including businesses, that are geared to helping young people establish positive self-esteem?

Family Planning Services

- What contraceptive information, counseling, and clinical services are available for adolescents? What is the number of adolescents (by age) who utilize these services each year?

- Can adolescents receive free family planning services in the community?

- How long does it take for an adolescent seeking a family planning appointment to receive care?

- Are contraceptive services for adolescents advertised in the community?

- How are teenagers assured of the confidentiality of services?

- Are condoms and other over-the-counter contraceptive methods made easily accessible in local pharmacies, drugstores, and other stores? Can adolescents readily purchase condoms at these locations? Can adolescents receive free condoms at other sites, such as clinics?

- What agencies sponsor family planning services in the community?

- Are there special efforts to reach young people with contraceptive information and/or care in schools, recreational settings, job training sites, etc.?

- What are the unmet needs in health services for adolescents, both male and female?

- What family planning is provided for children in foster care, both in foster family homes and in group home facilities?

For each of the family planning and family life education questions, specify each activity; number of participants, by age, race, and sex; access to services; outreach; and funding.

Media

- In terms of the adolescent audience in your community, rank the most popular media sources in your community, including television shows watched most often, most popular radio stations and radio programs reaching young people, and which newspapers are read.

- Have the media been used within the last two years to get across a pregnancy prevention message?

- If such a campaign was conducted, who sponsored the message? To whom was it targeted? What was the duration of the campaign? What type of media was used, and what did it accomplish? How were these findings measured?

Other Local, County, and State Efforts

- Has there been any public action within the last five years, on the local or state levels, to prevent adolescent pregnancy, such as the creation of a task force to study the impact of adolescent pregnancy in the community?

- Who has taken the lead in this effort, for example, governor, mayor, city council, community leaders, etc.?

- Have any private organizations or advocacy groups taken an active role in addressing the issue of adolescent pregnancy and pregnancy prevention? Specify the groups, their activities, their target population, and the outcomes of their efforts.

- Are there any public and/or private programs relating to pregnancy prevention operating within or associated with the schools? Within other community settings?

- Are there any public and/or private programs for employment training and placement for students who have dropped out or are on the verge of dropping out of school? Specify who the providers are, the type of training and jobs available, outreach and access to the program, numbers of participants by age, sex, and race/ethnicity, numbers of adolescents on waiting lists, numbers of adolescents who have been successfully placed in jobs, and funding sources of programs. Is there any coordination with school programs?

- What kinds of government-sponsored activities are available in the community, and who are the target groups?

- Is there any private sector involvement in the schools or other community sites? For example, mentoring programs, job "shadowing" or apprenticeship programs, grants to schools, summer placements, etc.?

- Are there any other school-initiated and/or school-based programs aimed at overall adolescent risk reduction and pregnancy prevention in particular?

- Are there Summer job training programs for youth, other federal, state, or local job training, or placement programs available for youths?

- Are there multi-service comprehensive programs that integrate all the services needed by adolescents? For example, sites where students can receive counseling, tutoring, recreation, and job training skills?

Questions for Providers, Key Community Decision-makers, and Gatekeepers

- What do you believe are the most critical problems or the greatest unmet needs facing youths in the community? What do you believe are the underlying causes? At the local level, what do you view as the biggest obstacle to solving each of these problems?

- What do you think should be done to resolve these barriers, and how are you involved in the solution of these problems?

- How concerned do you think the residents of the area are about each of these problems? Who are the most knowledgeable people in each of these problem areas?

- What local adolescent pregnancy prevention programs do you believe have been successful in your community? Why are they successful? What are your conclusions based on?

- Has there been any controversy surrounding the issue of adolescent pregnancy prevention in your community? What are the primary issues of controversy?

- What do you think needs to be done in your community to better address the problem of adolescent pregnancy prevention? What would you do first?

- What role can an agency like yours play in solving the problems you have described?

- What service gaps exist, and which factors create the greatest barriers to services?

- What networks, alliances, or relevant associations (formal and informal) already exist that target adolescents in the area of pregnancy prevention?

- Are there any other groups or key individuals who have not been identified and who could play an important role in reaching the target population?

- What groups or individuals might oppose these efforts? Why? How might your organization work with these programs in negotiating a consensus process?

- What intervention models currently in place in the community, aimed at your own target group or other at-need populations, have been successful in reaching at-risk populations?

- What previous efforts have been most successful? Least successful? (Note: You need to ascertain what factors have contributed to those successes and failures and whether these factors will be relevant to your efforts. A program may fail for organizational reasons — lack of appropriate leadership, insufficient community organization and planning efforts, lack of sufficient long-term funding and commitment to the problem, inappropriate staffing — or because needs were inadequately assessed in the planning stages of the program).

• What models exist in other communities, statewide or nationally, that have potential utility for your own target population? How would these models have to be adapted in order to meet the specific needs of your local community?

• What alternative strategies or models and efforts from other fields could be applied to the topic of adolescent pregnancy prevention; for example, model programs in the area of drug abuse prevention, or special efforts in the fields of education or social work that have relevance? How can each of these components be included as part of a community-wide plan directed at adolescent pregnancy prevention?

Worksheet 5-1

Needs Assessment Questions

Directions: On the lines below, list all questions you would like answered by your needs assessment.

Questions about the nature of the problem:

_Example: Which adolescent groups have the highest unintended pregnancy rates in the community?_____

_____

_____

_____

_____

Questions about existing resources:

_Example: What agencies provide family life education to schools?_____

_____

_____

_____

_____

Questions about successful programs previously implemented:

Example: _How well did your program meet the needs of young adolescents (<17) living in your community? What else could have been done to reach this target population?_____

_____

_____

_____

(and so on...)

Sources of Data for the Needs Assessment

Directions: In the first column enter your previously listed needs assessment questions. In the middle column note groups of people and other sources of data that might be able to provide you with relevant information. In the last column, list the methods of data collection you might use to answer each question. You may list more than one source of data or method of data collection for each question.

Needs Assessment Questions	Sources of Data	Methods of Data Collection
Example: *How well did your program meet the needs of community youth who are at risk of dropping out of school?*	▪ *Program records* ▪ *Follow-up survey of*	▪ *Review school records on each program participant* ▪ *Review last year's evaluation results* ▪ *Interview a group of past participants by telephone*

Worksheet 5-3

Needs Assessment Matrix

Name of Identified Agency	Services Provided	Number Reached	Referring Agencies (source of clients)	External Referrals	Collaborating Agencies	Community Needs Identified
Example: Anytown Community Youth Center	Recreational Education Tutoring On-site family life education Guest speakers Career speakers Sponsor community events	300 per month	Local schools, churches	Employment program Health clinics Family Planning Clinics Career counseling Volunteer opportunities in the community College-bound counseling	YMCA YWCA Anytown Health Department High School	Need similiar programs in other sites Need more on-site staff to expand program to younger adolescents Need ways to include parents and other family members Need better communication with agencies we refer our kids to

Chapter 6

Utilizing Needs Assessment Data To Create An Implementation Plan

The community needs-assessment survey will generate a tremendous amount of information and data. Using the information to establish service priorities for the coalition is the next important step in the planning process. The data become a valuable guide for developing a community-wide plan, helping you to decide which groups to target and what array of services to provide.

The program planning process requires a major commitment on the part of the coalition and the service providers of the community over an extended period of time. The process will challenge the community to:

- Reassess how the resources that are currently available can be used most effectively in meeting the needs of the target community;

- Assess what additional resources are needed and how best to utilize those resources;

- Determine what components of the community plan can be incrementally implemented in the community.

The plan becomes the guide for community action and evaluation. It documents what populations are most in need, what efforts are already underway, what service gaps exist in the community, and what possible directions the community-wide effort can take. It also describes the various activities the coalition will pursue over a period of time, usually three to five years. It should also include a proposed set of policy recommendations and specific steps to implement them.

This chapter discusses specific ways to develop an implementation plan based on the needs assessment findings. Many of the following examples are geared to family planning needs but are readily adaptable for planning other kinds of programs, which should be undertaken at the same time (such as programs for improving access to education, employment, and other life options).

Selecting Planning Areas

Many communities recognize that the number of people in need of services often exceeds the community's available resources. Thus, while all adolescents living in a community could benefit from a full array of coordinated services, specific high-risk populations require special action to ensure that they receive the necessary services. Communities have to weigh access issues for each component of the plan. For example, they may establish that family life education should be mandated for all children enrolled in public and private schools, but may elect to add a special health services program for high-risk adolescents whose lack of financial resources prevents them from seeking care. Or a coalition that is not in a position to plan brand new programs can ensure that existing support programs are made available to high-risk youth.

If the community you have chosen covers a whole city, a county or even a large neighborhood, it is important to subdivide it into manageable planning areas, so that services and programs will be within reach of the clients.

There are five approaches to the selection of planning areas:

1. Are there already service delivery districts for health, educational, and social services? If the plan is going to be broad-based and include each of these elements, it is important to use these service delivery districts as planning areas. For example, existing health planning areas or school districts could be the geographic reference areas.

2. Are there natural communities or neighborhoods that can serve as a basis for planning? Such boundaries may be difficult to establish without detailed research and often even local people have trouble defining the boundaries between one neighborhood and another.

3. Are there physical characteristics (such as state and county lines, rivers, freeways, etc. that can be used to delineate planning areas)?

4. Are there transportation networks which enable you to define areas?

5. Are there already a sizeable number of existing facilities providing youth services? If so, a combination of geographic and transportation approaches can be used in setting up "catchment areas" based on the number of potential clients to be served.

This method is biased toward facilities and services that are currently in place, and requires knowledge about current client loads.

In all instances, planning areas must incorporate census tract information, since the estimation of need is based on demographic data. Besides the census data, city hall or the department of health may have information broken down by census tract. Decisions can be made by mapping alternative schemes and totalling census tract figures to see if the districting plan is logical, fits in with other planning considerations, and is understandable to the local community. If planning areas have fewer than 500 young people, for example, they could be combined with contiguous areas and/or with other areas with similar characteristics. If areas have more than 5,000 young people in need, they may be divided.

Census data for the planning areas you have selected will provide much of the information you need, supplemented by local vital statistics, special census studies, regional planning data, or information from local commissions. These sources of data are also used to update information and to determine whether indicators such as the percentage of families living in poverty and births to adolescents have remained the same.

Defining The Target Population

The following steps can be used to calculate the number of adolescents at risk of an unintended pregnancy and in need of access to subsidized family planning care. Use a map of the geographic area(s) designated as planning areas, and pinpoint where the population in need of services resides, where services are available, and where gaps are likely to exist.

1. Estimate the number of female adolescents at potential risk of unintended pregnancy living in the selected planning area (females aged 12-14, 15-17, 18-19). If population figures are based solely on previous census data, increase or decrease this number by the estimated percentage of increase or decrease for your targeted area since the census year. Has the community experienced a new influx of residents? Has this influx altered the adolescent population figures? As new census data are available, note how much of an increase or decrease has occurred in the community during the past decade.

2. To estimate the number of medically dependent adolescent females of childbearing age, multiply the female teenage population number by the proportion of families with incomes below poverty. Poverty distributions are available from census data, as well as from county and city data books also published by the Bureau of the Census. If possible, obtain poverty estimates for the smaller areas you are studying, and follow the same procedure.

It is important to note that in terms of family planning care, adolescents of all income levels are often considered to be medically needy because their lack of personal income and their desire for confidential visits may well prevent them from using family income for care. Federal family planning Title X funding recognizes these potential barriers to care and thus offers services to adolescents at no charge or on a sliding scale.

3. If the community needs assessment did not document the incidence of teen sexual activity and contraceptive use, it is possible to use national data to project the number of youths in need of care. Based on special tabulations such as the 1983 National Longitudinal Survey of Youth by the Center for Human Resource Research, Ohio University (see Appendix 6–1), it is possible to make projections on the proportion of adolescents who are sexually active.

Based on these numbers and the age, sex, race, and ethnic composition of the community being studied, one can begin to compare the potential need (the number of adolescents at risk) against the number of sexually active adolescents being served through family planning clinics, making it possible to estimate the shortfall in family planning services (see Worksheet 6-1). For the purpose of estimating the amount of services needed by teenagers, for example for 15- to 17-year-olds, the minimum percentage of sexually active adolescents could be estimated to be between 20 and 50 percent. (See Appendix 6-1 for tables that can help you with this estimate.) It can also be assumed that at least one-third to one-half of sexually active teenagers will need subsidized family planning services (see data on poverty in Appendix 6-1). Use the data gathered through the needs assessment survey of family planning agencies to determine how wide the gap is between services provided and estimated need in the target community.

To make an assessment of the fit between the need for family planning services and the availability of services, it is necessary to analyze how many adolescents are already receiving care in the designated community. Remember that some adolescents who are using birth control will be impossible to document because they are using commercial over-the-counter methods and/or receiving private medical care.

As part of this assessment, it is important to take geographic proximity to services into account. Most agencies have information on the geographic area they serve, and each major family planning service provider, as well as those in related fields such as education and social services, should have been asked to provide detailed information on the estimated number of adolescents they serve, what services they provide, and the distance their clients travel to obtain services. Clients may then be broken down into two groups – those who live within a two-mile radius and those who live outside this area.

To assess the geographic proximity of services to the target population, list the locations of all available clinic sites and the numbers of adolescents they serve. (This

Worksheet 6-1

Anytown Family Planning Service Profile to Document Adolescents in Need of Family Planning Services

Total number of projected sexually active adolescents: _____

Total number served in fiscal year 1990: ‾ _____

Total unserved: _____

Percentage unserved: _____%

Family planning services in fiscal year 1990

- Hospitals providing family planning services (number): _____
- Number of adolescents served (ages): <15 ____, 15-17____,18-19 ____

Health Department providing family planning services Yes ☐ No ☐

- Number of Health Department locations providing family planning ____
- Number of adolescents served (ages): <15 ____, 15-17 ____,18-19 ____
- Number of Health Department locations not providing family planning___

Planned Parenthood affiliated services

- Number of locations for family planning services:_____
- Number of adolescents served (ages): <15 ___, 15-17 ___,18-19 ____

Other agency family planning services

- Number of locations for these services:_____
- Number of adolescents served (ages): <15 ___, 15-17 ___,18-19 ____

Total number family planning clinic locations:_____

Total number of adolescents served: _____

% by Hospital____% % by Planned Parenthood____%

% by Health Department_____% % by Other ____%

Fiscal resources to support services for adolescents

(Funding per agency, including source of funding)

Source of funding   Total Funding

_____   _____

_____   _____

_____   _____

                                                            Total _____

Note: Similar tables can also be used to calculate services needed to address school dropout problems, job training, and related concerns.

data should also be visually documented on your community map.) This network of agencies will most likely be the service backbone for the community plan. Assessing their capacity to fill the existing gap in services is a crucial step, one that can lead to the development of additional or alternative patterns for service delivery among existing agencies. This assessment of capacity will also help to determine whether new geographic sites should be utilized for providing care, including outreach, screening, health education, and referrals. As you review where agencies are located and consider where to plan alternative sites, it is also important to assess geographic proximity for the client. Ideally, 75 percent of clients using the service should be drawn from communities or neighborhoods closest to the clinic, preferably within two to five miles.

Because the availability of transportation plays a particularly important role in rural and suburban communities, it must be a major consideration in program planning. If transportation is less than adequate, efforts should be made to provide "one-stop" service centers. The lower density in rural areas, and the likelihood that distances will far exceed two miles may make it beneficial to use a travel time factor here instead of mileage factors in selecting service sites.

The following planning charts will be useful in compiling data from your needs assessment and applying it to specific target communities. This information will help the community assess:

- Whether current services are being utilized effectively;

- The expansion capacity of current services;

- Where additional services need to be placed;

- What additional financial and staff resources will be necessary.

Chart 6-1, Planning Overview, can be used to provide an overall picture for the community, based on summary information derived from Chart 6-2. The planning charts should reflect the primary objectives established by the community and should be developed for each major service. Examples in the next sections of this chapter show how to establish a plan aimed at meeting family planning needs within the target community.

Parallel planning should occur in meeting education, employment, and other life option objectives established by the coalition.

Chart 6-1

Planning Overview

1. Overall need (numbers of youth needing care)
   - Numbers of youth needing family planning (see Worksheet 6-1)
     (Add other identified coalition objectives as appropriate, for
     example, numbers of youth needing school remediation or job
     training programs.)

2. Current services and total of clients served (see Chart 6-2, Column #2)

3. Unmet need before plan (subtract #2 from #1)

4. Potential new clients at ongoing sessions (see Chart 6-2, Column #3)

5. Potential new clients at new sessions, old sites (see Chart 6-2, Column #4)

6. Potential new clients at new sessions, new sites (see Chart 6-2, Column #5)

7. Total potential new clients (add #4, #5, and #6)

8. Residual unmet need (subtract #7 from #3)

9. Total number of services needed for new clients at new sites (see Chart 6-2,
   Column #5)

10. Coalition priority rating where next services should be implemented (see
    Chart 6-2, Column #6)

Chart 6-2

Planning Areas
Expansion Potential of Existing Facilities

1	2		3		4		5		6
Agency	Current Services		Potential for new clients at ongoing sessions		Potential for new clients at new sessions at ongoing sites		Potential for new sessions at new sites		Coalition priority rating
	Total Clients	# of Sessions	Total Clients	# of Sessions	Total Clients	# of Sessions	Total Clients	# of Sessions	

Assessing the Expansion Potential of Existing Programs

There are a number of alternative ways to increase the number of youths reached by the network of services available in a community, including:

1. Increase the number of new clients being served at ongoing sessions in currently available sites through increasing efficiency of available services.

2. Serve additional clients at new additional sites.

3. Coordinate services with existing providers to assure equitable distribution of the same type of services throughout the community. Designate and delegate different organizations to perform specific tasks.

4. Expand the types and array of services current clients are receiving at each site.

Extending the kinds and quantity of services available for community youth requires a balanced assessment of whether the existing service delivery system can be increased by either reallocation of available resources and/or seeking additional resources. Inevitably, you will find some agencies already operating at a maximum with increasing waiting lists, while others remain under-utilized, often because of established eligibility requirements, location, or other barriers to care.

The first level of analysis is quantitative, as you determine the optimum capacity of all current and prospective facilities in each planning area. After this initial analysis is completed, a second level of qualitative analysis should be undertaken, allocating clients and identifying desirable locations for facilities. An approach for calculating staff time requirements is included in Appendix 6-3 at the end of this chapter.

To calculate client capacity for an existing program, compare the current number of clients served by the facility to its optimum capacity. If the difference is positive (+), the agency has the capacity to add new clients to its existing program. If the difference is negative (–), additional services are needed, perhaps through expansion of the program into new sessions. If funding requirements and the number of youths in need of services are extensive, the agency may need to reexamine how current services are being provided. For example, an educational tutoring program offering one-on-one attention could perhaps conduct group sessions in specific topic areas, such as math and English. Another option is to train administrative assistants to work closely with case managers and provide additional assistance with brokering of services. This allows case managers to provide care to additional clients, as well as more extensive counseling to their existing clients.

Another consideration is whether the physical space of the program can accommodate additional sessions. The staff must decide whether or not to establish additional sessions on the same site or to establish satellite sites to accommodate underserved areas. Satellite sites can often be established in other community agencies, particularly those that are already part of the coalition. In some situations, a "space exchange" or sharing (co-location) may be feasible for collaborating agencies. Sharing of space requires formal arrangements between agencies, as well as additional outreach, marketing, and advertising to inform potential users of the availability of services.

When planning new programs, one can use the experience of similar programs to estimate the numbers of clients that can be served and the numbers of sessions and staff required. In addition, the organizers must assess the amount of time it will require to implement the program once necessary resources are available. Already established programs in or outside the target community can often share their experience in establishing a new facility.

Setting Priorities for Facility Expansion

In setting priorities regarding which facilities to expand and/or to open, three qualitative factors must be considered in the following order of importance:

1. Integration of new efforts within the established network;

2. Location in relation to the concentration of youths in need of services;

3. Access to care, including convenience of transportation, hours, cost, and eligibility requirements.

The qualitative assessment requires that, working closely with the community, coalitions establish their primary goal. For example, the coalition should decide whether its primary goal is to establish programs in a wide array of agencies, to establish programs in the highest need areas first, or to establish programs that have increased accessibility. While financial and other resources may well dictate which of these goals is adopted first, communities must develop a consensus on where to place their focus initially, basing their decision on the completed needs assessment, agency interview information, maps, transportation information, and schedules.

Integration of New Efforts Within the Established Network

Assuming the highest priority is given to developing multi-pronged adolescent pregnancy prevention efforts within the already existing youth-serving system, a number of sites must be included in every plan, such as health facilities, schools, community-based or religious organizations, recreation sites, and job training sites.

In addition to sites, the components of the plan must be considered, including family life education, access to family planning services for sexually active adolescents, efforts at improving life options for youths by providing increased supports, and general education and employment efforts. For example, it may be unrealistic to plan a satellite family planning clinic in a job training site for youth, but it may be highly appropriate to incorporate a series of family life education sessions in existing training programs, to place a part-time family planning counselor on-site, and to provide initial family planning information, counseling, and referrals. Before such a program is established, however, it is important to consider whether it might be more rewarding to establish a program in an after-school recreation program reaching many more adolescents, at younger ages. In addition, one must consider the receptivity of the community to the development of these programs. It may be advisable to establish a worthwhile program that is perceived as less controversial as a means of setting a precedent and building trust within the community.

Timing is another consideration. It may be desirable to establish a priority system for introducing different programs over a five-year period, wherein, for example, the first two years are devoted to establishing an after-school recreation program, and a job-training program is introduced in year three or four. The plan must also consider how the role of existing staff can be expanded, perhaps with the help of continuing education.

It is not unusual in a community to find it easy to fund one project, while another that seems equally worthwhile is left unfunded. To compound matters, a program to which your coalition assigns a low priority score may receive sufficient funding to be implemented, while top priority programs go unsupported (see Chart 6-3). Priority ratings result from the community standards (see Chapter 4) and the overall priorities that communities establish for themselves. The community groups must then evaluate the circumstances and decide how to proceed, weighing matters of priority against fiscal and political reality.

The following example for Anytown (Chart 6-3) shows how to develop a system for establishing different components of a comprehensive adolescent pregnancy prevention program. This chart combines information gathered from the needs assessment in Chapter 5 (Currently Available Services and Community Sites) with the community standards and priorities established by the coalition in Chapter 4 (reflected in the Priority Area column and in the Ideal Community Standards column.) By establishing where both priorities and gaps exist within specific community sites, additional planning can occur. While few sites may be able to provide all three top program priorities – family life education, access to comprehensive family planning services, and improved life options – each community should aim to provide all three at one or more sites.

Location in Relation to Concentration(s) of Youths in Need

Is the planned facility near high density need areas? Are there other community services in the area that provide services to youths, but do not have a distinct adolescent pregnancy prevention focus?

Before rating facilities, each community must establish the appropriate numbers of youths they wish to serve, based on geographical boundaries, neighborhoods, etc.

Chart 6-3 **Priority Ratings for Anytown's Program Sites**

Priority Established by Coalition	Community Sites	Program Components	
		Ideal Community Standards	Currently Available
1	**Health**		
	Public Health clinics	1, 2	1, 2
	Neighborhood Health Centers	1, 2	1, 2
	Family Planning clinics	1, 2	1, 2
	Private Ob/Gyn, Pediatricians, and Family Practice providers	2	2
	Outpatient hospital departments	2	2
1	**Schools**		
	High schools	1, 2, 3, 4	1
	Middle schools	1, 3, 4	1
	Elementary schools	1, 3, 4	none
	School affiliated after-school programs	1, 2, 3	none
2	**Community-based Youth Serving Organizations and Recreation Sites**		
	National youth serving organizations	1, 2, 3	3
	Community recreation centers	1, 3	3
	Neighborhood youth programs	1, 2, 3	3
2	**Religious Congregations**		
	Parent-child communication workshops	1, 3	none
	Youth programs	1, 3	none
3	**Job Training**		
	Job apprenticeship programs	1, 4	4
	Job mentoring programs	3, 4	4
	Job training program for school dropouts	1, 2, 3, 4	4
	Summer training programs	1, 2, 3, 4	4

Program Components

1 = Family Life Education

2 = Access to family planning services, including referrals and direct services

3 = Preventive services to maximize use of existing education and employment programs and opportunities.

4 = Improved opportunities for academic and vocational education and employment.

For example:

Priority Established by Coalition	Geographic Location
1	Within a 2 mile radius – a maximum number of youths in need of adolescent pregnancy prevention services and no other programs available.
1	Within a 2 mile radius – a minimum number of agencies interested in integrating or strengthening their activities aimed at reducing unplanned pregnancy.
2	Beyond 2 mile radius – a maximum number of youths in need of adolescent pregnancy prevention services and no other programs available.
2	Beyond 2 mile radius – a minimum number of agencies interested in integrating or strengthening their activities aimed at reducing unplanned pregnancy.

Access to Care

Is the planned program or facility near reliable, inexpensive public transportation? Here is an example of transportation ratings:

Priority Established by Coalition	Available Transportation
1	Public – regularly scheduled; stops near facility, does not require transfer, reasonable costs.
2	Public – inconvenient; excessive trip costs or no transportation available.

While most plans will make an effort to implement all programs with a number 1 rating, there will be instances in which a choice must be made among several facilities. In these instances, location and transportation may become the determining factors. One should study the entire plan to be sure that the planned programs and sites cover the areas of intense need, and that the unmet need will be dramatically decreased. Before new sites are implemented, assess whether the available sites are functioning at capacity. Include in this assessment whether overlapping target areas are served by the available facilities.

Sample Plans

The following samples show how the Anytown coalition developed comprehensive, community-wide implementation plans. Although these plans will be undergoing changes as they are implemented, they become the basis for assessing community changes through time. Outlines of the plans, distributed to all participating partners, will help synchronize their efforts during the implementation phase.

Excerpts from Anytown's Adolescent Pregnancy Prevention Plan:
Family Life Education Component

Program Plan

Agency	Lead Agency: Anytown School District.
	Collaborating Agencies: Health Department and Planned Parenthood.
Goal	To provide comprehensive family life education for 14,000 students in the K-12 grades district wide.
Target Area	City-wide high schools will be targeted during Phase 1 (years 1 and 2) while middle schools and elementary schools will be reached during Phase 2 (years 3 and 4).

Overall Program

Design	When the full curriculum program is implemented, students will receive a comprehensive curriculum initiated in the elementary school and expanded and reinforced at the middle and high school levels. The curriculum will be taught at developmentally appropriate levels and will include the following:

- General health

- Anatomy, physiology, and reproduction

- Sexuality

- Family planning and reproductive health, including specific information on the consequences of teenage pregnancy

- Sexually transmitted diseases, including AIDS

- Life skills, including ways to strengthen self-esteem

- Sexual abuse prevention

- Tobacco, drug, and alcohol education

- Social/personal skills, including communication, interpersonal relationships, and decision-making

- The influence of the media and society on sex roles.

Administration: The program will be coordinated by the local school district, and a curriculum will be developed by a joint committee of school, parent, and community representatives. This committee will review all curriculum materials and provide guidance in implementation. Teacher training will be conducted throughout the school district, and a special coordinator will be designated at each school site to oversee the program components, arrange for outside speakers and agency participation, and monitor the quality of the program. Health educators from the health department and Planned Parenthood will be able to provide teacher training and team teach the family life education curriculum as it is implemented.

Budget: The current budget for family life education is $20,000, and is primarily devoted to the high school teaching program; an additional $45,000 is needed to expand the program as planned.

Case Management Services for At-risk Youth

Agency: Lead Agencies: Family Services Agency and School District.

Collaborating agencies: Social Services, Public Health Department, including substance abuse prevention and treatment programs, community recreation programs, and job training.

Goal: To provide services to a minimum of 400 adolescents deemed to be at high risk of school dropout and/or pregnancy.

Target Area: Middle schools and high schools in central and southeast regions of the city. Depending upon the success of the program, Phase 2 of the project will expand the program to the northeast region of the city.

Design: Adolescents identified as being on the verge of dropping out of school (e.g., experiencing a high degree of truancy, school failure, or other major difficulties with school), in trouble with the police, homeless, etc. will be referred to this program by school staff, health center staff, recreation staff, etc. A roving team of case managers will be available to school sites and other locations, including drug treatment centers, where adolescents may be reached. A complete educational and psychological assessment will be conducted at program entry, an individualized work plan will be established, and a case manager will follow each adolescent continuously for a minimum of two years. The case manager will also play an important role in brokering a variety of community agencies and services.

Administration: The program will be conducted by the Family Services Agency (fiscal agency) and the school district working collaboratively with a wide variety of community agencies that work with at-risk youths. A memorandum of agreement will be developed for each of the participating agencies, enabling the case manager to co-locate at each of the sites as appropriate, and also to facilitate referrals and follow-up.

Ten case managers, carrying a load of 40 adolescents each, will receive special training on working with at-risk youths who are still enrolled in school or who have recently dropped out of school. They will conduct case conferences with relevant agency and school personnel and follow up with their clients across different systems. At least half of the case managers will be regular school system employees whose job responsibilities have been revised and expanded.

Budget: The program will cost approximately $250,000, with one-half of the budget supported by the school system and one-fourth supported by the Family Services Agency through United Way funds. The remaining fourth will be supported through in-kind contributions by each of the participating agencies.

Structure for Coordinating Functions

To organize all parts of a multi-agency, community-wide program, a coordinating mechanism is essential. This function is performed by an overall coordinating organization which may not do the actual work but maintains responsibility for overseeing and organizing the activities of the participating agencies. This monitoring assures that there is no duplication of effort or unnecessary overlapping of functions, and that agencies are performing those functions for which they are best equipped. The lead agency, which oversaw the community planning process, may be the most appropriate choice to continue the same role in the implementation phase of the project. The coalition and the advisory board must review whether the lead agency has the requisite coordinating capacity.

Functions That
Can Be Performed
by a Community-
wide Coordinating
Agency or Group

1. Administration

   • Supervise specialized staff needed to implement plan.

   • Serve as a liaison among sponsoring agencies.

   • Encourage informal relationships between the coordinating organization and the community at large.

   • Develop formal relationships between the coordinating agency and health, education, social service, and community agency networks.

   • Work to modify participating agency policies in order to minimize barriers to providing care.

   • Coordinate all functions of community-wide program.

2. Planning and Development

   • Translate the plan into funding proposals, with special attention to the identification of sources for matching funds.

   • Negotiate with funding sources for grants.

   • Circulate the plan in the community to gain public support.

   • Find new sources of financial support for expansion of the program.

   • Negotiate reimbursements from state and federal programs, such as Medicaid.

   • Adapt plan for local conditions.

   • Alter plans over time as conditions change.

   • Organize local citizen planning bodies and advisory group to advise the coordinating group regarding future developments.

3. Data Collection and Evaluation:

   • Measure program utilization, using:

     – centralized automated record system for administrative efficiency within each agency,

– client tracking system from program to program,

– available service statistics for overall programs and for each component,

– records for outreach, recruitments, appointment and follow-up system.

- Measure program effectiveness, tracking:

  – new clients being served, as percentage of those with identified need,

  – percentage of youth continuing to participate in programs,

  – long-term trends in birth rates, school dropout, job placement and retention.

4. Staff Development:

- Recruitment and training of:

  – health care personnel,

  – community aides to work with different programs,

  – volunteers, including a Volunteer Services Bureau.

- In-service training for existing staff:

  – seminars, conferences, continuing education units, placement services, etc.

5. Education and Outreach:

- Designing and organizing an outreach program adapted to each of the participating agencies that will systematically identify and reach the target population. This may include:

  – central referral phone number, preferably with capacity to make appointments,

  – media campaign, which may include radio, television, newspapers, bus signs, and flyers.

- Develop interagency referral forms that can be easily used for providing both referrals and follow-up feedback to the referring agency.

- Work with a variety of community groups, including parent groups, voluntary agencies, business organizations, etc. to inform them about the scope and intent of the community group.

- Develop education programs for professionals and groups in the community regarding youth development and adolescent pregnancy prevention.

- Develop education programs for students enrolled in schools of medicine, nursing, social work, psychology and public health.

6. Inter-agency program coordination:

- Utilize staff for maximum efficiency, including sharing of specialized personnel.

- Shift client flow from crowded facilities to new facilities which continue to be convenient to clients.

- Introduce new approaches, information, and potential models as they become available.

- Develop referral mechanisms for agencies that are not participating in the coalition.

Organizational Structures

In selecting the appropriate agency to coordinate the implementation, the coalition must consider the following questions:

1. Should the lead agency continue to be the coordinating agency?

2. Does the community need a different, independent and/or more neutral coordinating agency?

3. Should a new organization or entity be established if none exists in the community?

4. Is there an agency that is already providing a large number of services in the community, and that is best constituted to perform these functions?

One criterion for selection is the magnitude of administrative responsibility that the agency would take on as compared to the responsibility it now has. How does its current budget compare with the overall additional funds estimated for the entire program? A small agency may feel overwhelmed by the added responsibility of coordinating a full community project, while a larger agency may already have in place many of the needed administrative components. A second criterion is the adaptability of the present staffing patterns of the potential coordinating agency.

Charts 6-4 and 6-5 display different kinds of models that communities may consider adopting. Chart 6-4 shows the use of a coordinating agency or group whose sole function is to provide coordination in implementing the plan, while Chart 6-5 shows how coordination for each component would occur within the agency designated as the lead agency for that component. Other organizational structures may be adapted, depending upon the size of the community, the network of participating agencies, the kinds of agencies participating in the community-wide plan, and the availability of resources.

Chart 6-4

Coordinating Organization Structure: Separate Coalition Model, Divided Functions by Organization

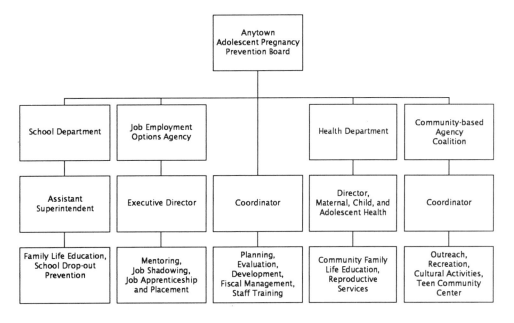

Chart 6-5

Coordinating Organization Structure: Separate Coalition Model

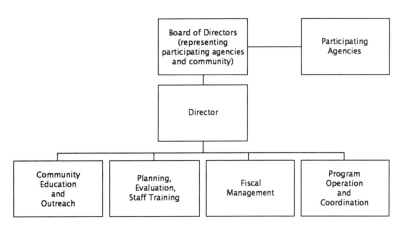

The Implementation Plan

By the time the community planning process has been completed, your coalition has come to recognize that to address the complex challenge of preventing adolescent pregnancy, multiple strategies will be required. The strategies and tactics of an implementation plan will identify who is going to do what, and when and how they will do it. The plan should specify measurable objectives and attainable goals. It should also describe accountability measures to assure achievement of these objectives and goals. These critical issues may test the trust and confidence built thus far in the collaborative process, but their avoidance will only create difficulties later on. Participating organizations should realize that through collaboration they are extending their own organization's efforts, rather than losing their autonomy.

Ideally, when the collaborative plan is fully developed, member organizations will recognize its goals and objectives as being consistent with their own goals and objectives.

The planning process should encourage maximum involvement of agencies in the plan's implementation. As the plan emerges, agencies will review, discuss, modify, and endorse it, identifying those areas in which they will provide leadership and resources, either individually or collaboratively. More than likely, tasks will be identified that individual agencies or small groupings of agencies can take on as their own. It is critical that these commitments be recorded in the plan. The coalition's adoption of a plan of action must be sensitive to the internal decision-making process that individual organizations must go through before they endorse the plan. Adoption of the plan, when all organizations have endorsed it, should be brought to the attention of the community at large, with an emphasis on collaboration among member agencies.

Gaining Community Support

Upon determining the community's needs, one of the first tasks of the coalition will be to formulate an effort to gain support among community residents, particularly adolescents and their parents, whom the program is designed to serve.

Begin by developing a statement of the needs assessment findings, developed according to the guidelines in Chapter 5. Remember to translate your findings into manageable, informative documents that can be used for building community support. Brief documents that visually summarize your findings become a powerful tool. For example, maps may be used to illustrate the locations of areas with a high incidence of adolescent births, low-birthweight babies, dropout rates, youth unemployment rates, etc. as well as potential locations of projected programs. Another possible way to communicate your findings is to show the number of adolescent births over the past ten years, or the effect of different kinds of educational interventions and their impact on school dropout rates. You may also want to select salient quotes to support the data you present. All this information must be blended into a statement which clearly spells out a message leading to action, including recommendations for solutions.

In order to build community support, recommendations that emerge from the coalition's study must be stated in manageable terms. Conditions such as poverty and unemployment, which are at the root of many social problems, are so global in nature that it becomes difficult to establish a set of specific recommendations to respond to them, and the chances for immediate change are limited. Generate a list of problems that are amenable to change and that will become the focus of your efforts, such as the high incidence of school dropout, or the need for additional recreational and after-school programs. Resolving some of these issues will begin to have some impact on the underlying issues affecting the community.

Formulating Goals and Objectives

Recommendations for implementing a new set of community strategies may take different forms (see example in Appendix 6-2). Your coalition may wish to develop specific goals, objectives, and action plans for each identified problem or cluster of problems. Throughout the planning process, the coalition must return to the community standards that represent the overall goals on which the coalition built its consensus.

It is helpful to proceed as follows:

1. Write objectives with specific projected timelines.

2. Outline specific activities or strategies to accomplish the established goals and objectives.

3. Identify resources needed to carry out activities (both additional financial support and available personnel and other resources).

4. Monitor and evaluate progress toward meeting the proposed goals and objectives.

Remember, an objective describes what actions must take place before a goal is achieved. A well-written objective contains detailed information. It tells you:

• Who will do it,

• What they will do,

• Why they will do it,

• When they will do it,

• Where and how the objective will be accomplished.

You may have already developed a preliminary set of goals, as your coalition was becoming established. Now that you have collected your needs assessment data, review those goals and evaluate whether they continue to be appropriate. Depending upon the array of services a community already has in place, you may find that the major focus of your plan will be in the coordination of current efforts into a more organized and extended community-wide effort. In communities where major gaps exist in services, the plan may focus on building financial and community support.

While some of the goal-setting process occurs before the needs assessment data are collected, much of the data you have collected will help either validate the original set of goals or raise a different set of goals. Another reason for developing community goals is to establish the ideal toward which the community strives.

At their core, strategies for implementing a community-wide adolescent pregnancy prevention plan should include the following components:

1. Coordination of Services Among Community Programs

Agencies can increase their level of effectiveness by working in conjunction with other programs to assure a better coordinated system of care. For example, agencies can establish formal exchanges of information and referral to increase the level of direct services, and improve access to care. They can also establish multi-service sites where several agencies can provide their services in a site convenient for youths and their families. In settings where this is not possible, consider co-location (placement of one agency's staff within another program) so that entry into other systems can be facilitated. For example, an eligibility worker or youth employment counselor placed in a school setting can be responsible for much initial completion of forms, recruitment, and referral. In addition, a relationship can be established between the youth and the provider that then can be extended into the "home base" of the agency sponsoring that service provider.

It is important to review the current activities of a variety of programs and their target populations in order to assess whether there is any duplication or inappropriate overlap between programs and targeted geographic regions. For example, community health educators representing different agencies may decide that instead of working in the same school, they should continue their education focus in separate locations, moving to schools that are in need of programs, but which have received less agency attention.

The community-wide plan will have a variety of objectives, from implementing specific new programs that target specific at-risk youths, to developing a comprehensive educational campaign reaching through all sectors of the community. In addition, improving coordination of services and the overall quality of care will most likely be among the objectives. For example, coordinating family life education efforts within a community (to ensure that young people receive a core set of information and that both in-school and out-of-school youth are reached) could require that parallel agencies work toward a shared goal. Agencies could work together to ensure that youths receive a comprehensive array of services, including health and family life education, school enrichment and remediation, monitoring, job preparation, and job training options, as well as cultural and recreational activities. Thus, the same community plan may encompass categorical and comprehensive programs.

It is important to recognize that while coordination efforts increase the efficient use of available resources, the process of coordination is time- and staff- intensive for all participating agencies. Thus, adequate staff support is crucial for effective program coordination.

2. Program Planning and Development

A community-wide plan aims at providing youths with a comprehensive array of services and opportunities geared to increasing the level of motivation necessary to delay an initial pregnancy. Chart 6-6 illustrates the components of Anytown's comprehensive community-wide effort to reduce its teenage pregnancy rate.

Chart 6-6

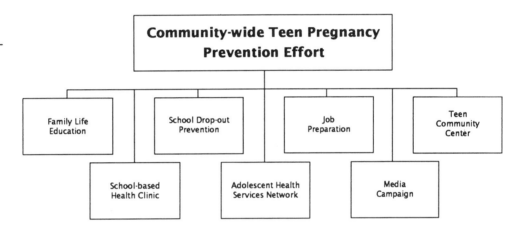

3. Community Awareness and Commitment to Community-based Adolescent Pregnancy Prevention Efforts

It is important that the broader community be made aware of the way that adolescent pregnancy impacts the greater community, and of alternative options for addressing the problem, including what models exist that could be adapted to meet the needs of the community's youth. Organizing the community to help your coalition find the necessary funding is one way that the community can gain ownership of the problem and its solution.

A full community education campaign should begin once the coalition and the agencies it represents are prepared to present their findings and discuss recommendations. A variety of educational approaches will be needed to reach a number of audiences, from parents, religious leaders and school personnel to elected officials. It is also important to assess whether adolescent pregnancy prevention is perceived to be a major problem as compared to other community issues, such as drug abuse and school dropout. The educational effort should clearly delineate the strong inter-relationships between these other pressing concerns and the topic of adolescent pregnancy prevention. Also, your needs assessment should have documented how the perceptions of the community regarding the problem of adolescent pregnancy compare to the data you have collected on the incidence of these problems. This contrast will often guide the educational effort.

4. Coordination of Funding

Although new monies may be needed to establish components of the community-wide strategy, many of these efforts can probably be implemented with available funding. However, it is important to review whether reallocation of available funding may contribute to increasing prevention efforts, as funds from several agencies may be pooled to support a new program effort. For example, an individual agency that may not be able to afford to hire a full-time youth coordinator may be able to fund 40 percent of the salary, and other community agencies working with the same youth population may be able to fund the rest, particularly if the coordinator will refer youths to their own programs.

Summary

Upon completion of the needs assessment the next critical stage of the coalition's work begins: creating an implementation plan. The information generated through the needs assessment must now be utilized to determine the target population, and the efforts that are already underway to serve them. The needs assessment serves as a mechanism to identify service gaps as well as to develop strategies to address existing needs. The implementation plan outlines the specific activities the coalition intends to undertake during specified time periods. This formal plan becomes the coalition's guide throughout the implementation and evaluation stages of its work.

The initial steps leading to the final plan include: selecting planning areas, defining the target population, assessing the expansion potential of existing programs, and setting priorities for facility expansion. All these steps require the full cooperation and involvement of the coalition members so that they feel it represents their goals and objectives. It is also imperative that they demonstrate a commitment to take part in the tasks to be undertaken. The sample plan and other sample material included in this chapter are designed to assist communities in designing their own plans.

Appendix 6-1

Data on Sexual Activity

Cumulative Sexual Activity by Age, Sex, Race, and Ethnicity

	Age	Sexually Active Male	Female		Age	Sexually Active Male	Female
Total	15	16.6%	5.4%	**Black**	15	42.4%	9.7%
	16	28.7	12.6		16	59.6	20.1
	17	47.9	27.1		17	77.3	39.5
	18	64.0	44.0		18	85.6	59.4
	19	77.6	62.9		19	92.2	77.0
	20	83.0	73.6		20	93.9	84.7
	(N)	(4,657)	(4,648)		(N)	(1,146)	(1,157)
White	15	12.1%	4.7%	**Hispanic**	15	19.3%	4.3%
	16	23.3	11.3	*(may be of*	16	32.0	11.2
	17	42.8	25.2	*any race)*	17	49.7	23.7
	18	60.1	41.6		18	67.1	40.2
	19	75.0	60.8		19	78.5	58.6
	20	81.1	72.0		20	84.2	69.5
	(N)	(2,828)	(2,788)		(N)	(683)	(703)

Source: Special tabulations from the 1983 National Longitudinal Survey of Youth, Center for Human Resource Research, Ohio University

Percent Sexually Active, by Age, Ethnicity, Region, and Poverty Status Among Unmarried Teenagers

Age	Poverty Status	Region	White & Others	Black
15-17	<150% poverty	(NE) North East	32.4	53.5
		(NC) North Central	44.0	49.6
		(S) South	47.6	55.7
		(W) West	47.4	61.0
	150-249% poverty	NE	20.3	37.4
		NC	29.2	33.9
		S	32.2	39.5
		W	32.1	44.5
	250%+ poverty	NE	13.5	26.6
		NC	20.1	23.9
		S	22.5	28.4
		W	22.4	32.6
18-19	<150% poverty	NE	55.6	85.8
		NC	67.9	83.1
		S	71.4	87.2
		W	71.2	90.2
	150-249% poverty	NE	39.2	73.0
		NC	51.5	69.5
		S	55.2	74.9
		W	54.9	79.2
	250%+ poverty	NE	43.0	76.5
		NC	55.5	73.2
		S	59.3	78.3
		W	59.1	82.3

Source: The Alan Guttmacher Institute. Estimates based on 1982 National Survey of Family Growth data with an adjustment of an increase of seven percent in the proportion of sexually active between 1982 and 1987.

Appendix 6-2

Primary Goals and Strategies

Example

Anytown Comprehensive Adolescent Pregnancy Prevention Plan

Phase I and Phase II

Goals

1. To reduce the incidence of unintended adolescent pregnancy.

2. To increase the number of adolescents who delay having their first birth until they have earned a high school diploma.

3. To develop a comprehensive community-wide policy that addresses the complex and multifaceted problem of teenage pregnancy and childbearing and supports the implementation of a variety of interventions aimed at reducing the problem.

4. To implement an integrated and coordinated system of care delivery.

Specific Strategies: Phase I

1. Establish a community-wide advisory council consisting of representatives of city agencies, local and community coalitions, parents, and teenagers – ethnically, racially, economically, and geographically diverse – to develop and monitor policy, and to advise the mayor and the city council on adolescent pregnancy prevention.

2. Commit financial and political support to primary prevention efforts, including family life education, while providing access to reproductive health care. Seek additional funding in order to meet the needs of the targeted population, and upgrade the delivery of family planning services to sexually active teens.

3. Educate the general public about the impact of teenage pregnancy, childbearing and parenting in the community, and about the value of postponing first pregnancies until after adolescence.

4. Involve both female and male teenagers in developing strategies that target their peers.

Phase II

5. Expand the role of males in preventing adolescent pregnancy by actively involving them in deciding whether or not to be sexually active, in becoming committed to using contraceptives if they are so, and in being aware of the consequences of pregnancy and parenthood.

6. Involve parents in the formulation of policies in the area of adolescent pregnancy prevention, and in the coordination of services at the community level.

7. Implement a comprehensive health care plan for teenagers, which includes access to reproductive health services.

8. Support the development of community-based health and social services for teenagers, particularly school-linked services.

9. Inform young people of available health services in their communities and teach them how to be effective health consumers, including information on when it is appropriate to seek care.

10. Provide student support services through schools in order to help teenagers successfully complete their education.

Appendix 6-3

Calculating Staff Time Requirements

*B*ased on previous program experience, it is important to make calculations regarding the amount of time required to serve adolescents, in order to estimate the optimum number of youths that can be served by a single program. It is also important to assess how many new adolescents an agency can serve while maintaining ongoing relationships with established clients. Reviewing patterns of program use, including how many new clients and how many returning clients were served in the previous year, assess the level of client "retention" the program has and how much potential room for expansion exists. To get an estimate of how much staff time and client time is needed per visit, use the following chart, which is based on a case management program model that integrates school remediation activities and counseling. Estimated staff time will depend on how many of the following components are in place.

Estimated Staff Time and Client Time Per Patient Visit

Staff Required	New Clients		Established Clients		Staff Functions
	Staff Time (in minutes)	Client Time	Staff Time (in minutes)	Client Time	
Social Worker	60	45	15	15	• Conducts client assessment and follow-up monthly • Develops individual plan • Provides direct counseling services • Provides referral and brokering services • Maintains and updates records

Staff Required	New Clients		Established Clients		Staff Functions
	Staff Time *(in minutes)*	Client Time	Staff Time *(in minutes)*	Client Time	
Educational Specialist	60	45	30	15	▪ Conducts educational assessments ▪ Develops individual learning plan ▪ Supervises tutors ▪ Monitors student progress
Tutor	45	30	45	30	▪ Provides private tutoring/ mentoring ▪ Maintains educational objectives ▪ Attends case conferences
Health Educator	15	15 *(individual)*	15	15	▪ Gives individual/group sessions
	45	45 *(group)*	45	45	▪ Coordinates instruction with tutor and case manager
(plus preparation, 2 hours)					
Clerk	15	5	15	5	▪ Sets up new appointments ▪ Arranges referrals, and documents whether client followed up with appointment

1. Total staff time for established clients:_____

2. Total staff time for new clients:_____

3. Total direct client time for established clients:_____

4. Total direct time for new clients:_____

5. Total time per client:_____

Chapter 7

Implementing Community Strategies

*W*hen the planning process has resulted in a community implementation plan, then comes the challenge of acting on it. This chapter focuses on two primary implementation issues: how to maintain a viable coalition, and how to maintain a funding base to continue the efforts of the coalition.

Organizing the community to implement the strategies is the first step under the leadership of an implementation committee. A variety of approaches will be necessary to work with and educate the community on potential alternatives. Different strategies will be required for different community groups. For example, providing information to parents and school personnel on the issue of adolescent pregnancy and pregnancy prevention should not occur until a mechanism is established or a system is in place to respond to their concerns.

Through the process of building the coalition and conducting the needs assessment, you will have reached and educated many influential individuals and organizations in the community. You may have already identified existing networks and committees designed to address youth issues. These can become part of the implementation network that will assist in bringing the plan to fruition. In exchange, the coalition may need to join other youth-related efforts in order to combine the networks.

The Implementation Committee

An implementation committee will be valuable in identifying barriers, and assessing what aspects of the plan may be particularly difficult to implement. For example, you may consider at first that adopting a comprehensive K-12th grade family life education program will be a priority within your community's plan. However, after members of the implementation committee review what programs are already in place and the level of community acceptance of (or resistance to) the program, you may decide to build on your current program incrementally, rather than imposing a whole new one, so that the transition can go smoothly. It is preferable to address potential barriers rather than avoid them. Once they are addressed, it is possible to take specific steps to deal with those barriers, and find the areas of common agreement that will allow you to implement change.

The implementation committee can be made up of advisory board members, representatives of the lead agency, coalition members, and others who have a role to play. Representatives from each participating organization should take the implementation plan to their respective organizations for review and approval before the committee's work can proceed.

Establishing a Time Line

As you develop your series of objectives, you will need to develop a feasible time line. Review the following series of questions as you develop this component of your plan:

1. What critical tasks need to be accomplished?

2. What are the critical dates? For example, when do the tasks have to be accomplished in order to meet the projected implementation deadlines?

3. What other interim tasks have to be accomplished in order for the community-wide plan to be implemented?

Strengthening Collaboration

The community-wide program proposed in this book assumes that agencies participating in the coalition have begun to recognize the advantages of working together. It also implies that this attitude is shared, not only at the management level, but also at the direct service provider level. Having agency staff meet with other agency staff to foster opportunities for the exchange of existing information is crucial. It is through these exchanges of information that obstacles to coordination can be identified, and solutions developed (Rossi, Gilmartin, Dayton, 1982). A useful technique to overcome potential barriers is force field analysis. Appendix 7-1 illustrates the use of this method.

Before you can fully implement your program, verify that all member organizations are aware of and support the coalition's implementation plan. Producing a sense of ownership may be time consuming, but it is imperative for the success of your program. It is also important that each individual organizational representative is prepared to carry out his or her assigned responsibilities for implementing the plan in an efficient and timely manner. If necessary, appropriate training and technical assistance should be provided to assist coalition members. The coalition's collaborative plan is not intended to replace, duplicate, or compete with activities of the member organizations: it is intended to ensure that member organizations, acting individually or in small collaborative groupings, take responsibility for designated portions of the coalition's plan and be accountable to the coalition for their accomplishment.

In order for the collaboration to continue, it is necessary to:

1. Continue communication with the leadership of member agencies to assure that the coalition keeps the commitment of its members.

2. Consider working towards greater levels of commitment and standards of participation from member organizations, if this is necessary.

3. See the coalition as an ongoing process, always exploring new ideas and evaluating its own successes, failures, and capacity to provide a means for effective action.

Key ingredients for a successful working collaboration were outlined by Dunkle and Nash (1989). The collaborative relationship is identified with the following characteristics:

- It is legitimized by formal action of the boards of participating agencies and by regular participation in the collaborative decision-making process by high-level agency representatives.

- It has an established structure (operating procedures, officers, committees, management systems, planning processes, and identified accountabilities).

- It involves the widest possible range of local, voluntary, community and public agencies.

- It has mutually defined and accepted goals and objectives, based on a needs assessment; an action plan with activities to which individual agencies identify and commit their specific skills and resources; a mechanism for influencing community attitudes; public-policy funding; and service decisions through ongoing community education and advocacy efforts.

- It includes procedures for continuing skills development and capacity-building among member organizations.

- It has established linkages with appropriate public agencies and elected officials, and maintains continuing dialogue.

Implementing Interagency Coordination

An important technique for increasing the coalition's effectiveness is to facilitate interagency coordination, both for agencies that have common goals and for those that complement each other's missions. Interagency coordination is briefly defined as the collaboration of people from two or more agencies, working together to improve services to clients. Typically each agency operates under a distinct legal mandate and funding source, with its own administrative structure, geographical boundaries, and specific objectives. Although some agencies have informal interactions, it is a rare administrator who can provide real rewards that encourage wide adoption of formal interagency structures. However, this picture is changing, and many federal and state funded programs are beginning to require collaborations.

There are a number of ways that agencies working in related areas can coordinate with one another, without undue expense or difficulty, to their clients' benefit and their own, including:

- Establishing cross-referral networks,

- Developing joint goals and objectives,

- Providing case consultation, joint intake and assessment, and co-location,

- Joint gathering of data and program information,

- Joint program operation.

Advantages of interagency coordination are:

- Improved staff effectiveness — coordination can help make available to agencies the skills and knowledge of each others' staff, new equipment and facilities, and new services available to their clients;

- Improved accessibility for clients, who will learn more about available services;

- Reduced fragmentation of services, which will streamline bureaucratic require-ments for clients and facilitate each client's treatment as a whole person rather than seeing clients as a collection of unrelated problems;

- Greater efficiency in delivering more services for the same money or the same services for less money, through economies of scale, reduction of duplication, and improved cost-benefit ratios;

- Improved public image through greater efficiency and reduced duplication of efforts (Rossi, Gilmartin, and Dayton, 1982).

Exploring Outside Resources

Implementing a community's strategic plan will require a variety of financial re-sources, including new funding and/or reallocation of existing support. A number of resources are available to communities from a wide array of sources. Potential re-sources within communities include:

- **Local governing bodies.** Local officials can provide support for interagency coordination by 1) directly funding pilot projects using locally generated or locally controlled monies; 2) indirectly supporting cooperative efforts through reallocation of the budgets of county agencies; or 3) writing letters of support to assist in securing funds elsewhere.

- **Private interest groups and service organizations.** Chambers of Commerce, Lion's Clubs, Rotary Clubs, and many other civic service groups have been known to raise money for interagency efforts. They can also help in securing funding elsewhere. You might seek volunteer assistance to work on this effort. Sometimes other community agencies involved in cooperative planning are willing to help coalition efforts.

- **Businesses and industries.** Representatives of local businesses and industries may be persuaded to provide money, in-kind contributions, political support, job-development programs, and help in attracting other businesses in accomplishing the goals of the coalition.

Resources at the state and federal levels include:

- **Information for local-level planning.** Information for planning is often available for the asking; it can be supplemented by canvassing local data sources and small scale data gathering efforts supported by the local agency or community resources.

- **Technical assistance,** available for many geographical areas and types of agencies. Technical assistance providers represent important links to well-intentioned state and federal programs, and working with them may increase the chances of receiving state and federal support for cooperative ventures.

- **Grant and contract monies.** Many agencies are interested in funding efforts geared to supporting interagency coordination among local service providers.

Initiating Interagency Activities

The overall theme of the plan is to increase the level and amount of coordination that occurs on behalf of young people. It is important that agency representatives know enough about organizations to determine what kind of coordinated effort is possible. While some agencies may naturally lend themselves to close joint efforts, other less traditional collaborations can be explored. For example, community youth clubs could develop a referral relationship with family planning providers to help in identifying clients in need of care. These relationships must be close and ongoing if they are expected to work. Referral mechanisms may be only one of the many joint efforts that can be developed, including sponsoring workshops for parents and children, training agency staff, providing mentors, developing job shadowing positions, etc. Information in Table 7-1 has been adapted from a chart developed by Rossi, Gilmartin, and Dayton

(1982), and is an important check list for agency personnel who are exploring what their combined roles might entail.

Another important exercise is to assess what benefits exist for agencies that do collaborate. For example, they may become more efficient, expand available resources, and increase the effectiveness of agency administrators. This list will vary from agency to agency, as collaboration is a two-way street. Worksheet 7-1 outlines a checklist that can aid in assessing resources that become available through a collaborative process.

Fostering Cooperation

Interagency coordination requires a certain level of trust. Agency personnel must be given an opportunity to identify agencies with whom they share potential clients and with whom they have a good agency match. The most promising areas for initial exploration between agencies will be those in which a joint effort is plainly beneficial to both programs. If the agencies have never worked together before, it may be helpful for them to consider a joint pilot project initially, rather than a complex project that might overwhelm both agencies. Throughout this period, benefits to both agencies need to be clearly identified so that each agency has a stake in the relationship. Responsibilities should be structured so that each organization is carrying enough of the load to demonstrate commitment, and to play an active role in accomplishing joint objectives (Rossi, Gilmartin, Dayton, 1982).

Agency administrators should make the initial contact, and bring in other staff members when it is feasible. This is particularly crucial during the planning phase, so that any staff members' doubts regarding the new interagency relationships can be resolved.

The community-wide plan is an excellent focus point for efforts at initiating communication among programs, and exploring ways that interagency links can be established and joint efforts developed. Face-to-face meetings of agency staff allow them to become acquainted, ask questions, and acquire detailed information.

It is also possible that a variety of factors may discourage communication. For example, an agency may be operating under a crisis mode resulting from decreasing budgets, cutbacks in staff, and new community needs. Or it may experience staff inflexibility in adapting to new situations, turfmanship, bureaucracy, and conflicting interests among competing demands. There are several ways to overcome these problems:

• Recognize the existence of barriers. Prepare to address obstacles and determine why they exist.

• Focus on the overriding objective of meeting the needs of clients and on the intent

What Do You Know About Other Agencies?

Use this worksheet to help you evaluate your knowledge of each agency with which you plan to work on the implementation plan.

	No Knowledge	Some Understanding	Complete Information
1. The agency's main goal or mission	☐	☐	☐
2. The authority or legislation under which it operates (if any)	☐	☐	☐
3. The sources and amount of agency funding	☐	☐	☐
4. The agency administration	☐	☐	☐
5. The eligibility requirements for clients (if any)	☐	☐	☐
6. The approximate number of clients served annually	☐	☐	☐
7. The main services offered	☐	☐	☐
8. The expertise represented on staff	☐	☐	☐
9. The facilities and equipment the agency has	☐	☐	☐
10. Names, titles held, and telephone numbers of agency personnel	☐	☐	☐
11. Current activities, including participation in interagency cooperative projects	☐	☐	☐

of the agencies. Demonstrate how interagency coordination can improve the numbers of clients reached and the quality of care they receive, as well as how this increased efficiency is to the advantage of the organization.

- Identify key allies within each agency who can help get things done. Policy-making groups and advisory boards that oversee public and private agencies are also useful constituents in gaining support for coordination. Involve these groups early in the process as they often have the responsibility of approving interagency proposals in advance.

- Create structures within each agency that reward staff for fostering coordination efforts.

The coalition's advisory group can coordinate an interagency task force to implement the whole plan, or it may choose to identify task forces to work on specific goals, bringing together a number of agencies. For example, if a major goal of the adolescent pregnancy prevention plan is to increase the numbers of students who graduate from school, then representatives from schools, parent groups, community-based organizations, job training programs and businesses could come together as a task force to formulate a plan. Ideally the group would include all potentially interested parties, have no more that twelve to fifteen representatives working together, have designated individual responsibilities, and develop realistic goals and objectives. Although final authority for implementation of the objectives would remain with the sponsoring agency, it would be important for these representatives to be fully committed to the process, and to implementing changes within their agencies or organizations as a result.

Formal Agreements

The need for some formal agreement stating the nature and purposes of working arrangements agreed upon by two or more agencies varies from community to community. There are certain advantages to drawing up these memoranda of agreement (MOAs) or memoranda of understanding (MOUs) as they establish the roles and responsibilities for each cooperating agency in the effort to implement a common set of coordinating objectives. These agreements:

- Force the agencies to define their objectives and roles,

- Specify who is to take responsibility for managing and evaluating joint activities,

- Provide a reference point when problems arise,

- Can be modified easily when changes take place because they are not legally binding,

- Usually can be agreed upon without formal approval by the agencies' funding sources,

- Represent an initial symbol of trust and intended cooperation among the agencies involved.

Descriptions of the scope of services to be coordinated and the responsibilities of the two or more cooperating agencies would also be included in the agreement. This process should help to achieve coordination through the development of a strong sense of common purpose.

*Meeting Client
Needs Through
Effective Referrals*

A common way for agencies to work together is through the process of making referrals to one another. As the community begins implementing the community-wide strategies, agencies will need to ask: 1) how effective are currently existing referral systems; and 2) what agencies that are currently not participating in this network should be involved in providing referrals? Important questions to address are:

• In how many cases are the appropriate number of clients being referred, and are these clients eligible for the services provided by the receiving agencies?

• Are the numbers of clients who are being cross-referred appropriate to the client load of the receiving agencies?

• Are agencies monitoring referrals? Are good records maintained?

• Are there ways that agencies can improve the effectiveness of referrals?

• How many of these agencies have two-way referrals?

To establish a formal cross-referral network, create a multi-agency directory or brochure that will help agencies maintain records of the services available through other agencies and organizations in the community. These documents are especially useful when one is orienting staff to the requirements of other agencies, provided they are regularly updated to reflect changes in regulations or procedures and are supplemented by direct contact among agency staff. As you are implementing the community plan, conduct regular meetings of interagency staff, and work with them to implement record-keeping systems for referrals (including acknowledgment of each referral received).

*Ways to Decrease
Service
Fragmentation*

As the community implements the activities outlined in the plan, coordination problems may emerge which affect all service delivery.

Four approaches have been identified by Rossi, et al. (1982) that can be used to decrease service fragmentation:

• **Case consultation** involves staff from one agency consulting with staff from another agency for information that can assist providers to improve the care they deliver. It may include assessing whether the client's needs are being met and what services the mutual client is already receiving.

• **Client conferences** are more formal than case consultations; staff from two or more agencies meet to discuss the needs of all the clients they have in common.

• **Client teams** are made up of staff from two or more agencies who coordinate their activities to meet the needs of a number of clients, through continuous and systematic interaction. This can make the intake process more efficient. Groups of clients can initially meet with the team, rather than going from one agency to the next, to reduce fragmentation and duplication of services. Clients can then deal with the same team over time. Client teams usually interact on a regular basis with their clients. Registration information, eligibility requirements, paperwork, and intake procedures are greatly facilitated, and the clients can avoid multiple visits. Teams should be together at least once a week in the same office to facilitate follow-up.

- **Case Management** allows case managers from one agency to have responsibility for coordinating services provided by several agencies. Case managers provide direct services and assist clients by brokering a variety of services, often facilitating their entry into each program. The knowledge and efforts of case managers cross agency boundaries, since their responsibility is to follow clients across systems. Thus, interagency coordination is focused on one primary anchor.

Assessing how many collaborating agencies are involved in each of these approaches is important in increasing the level of interagency coordination necessary for implementing the overall community plan.

Ways to Increase Accessibility of Client Services

There are four approaches that may greatly facilitate outreach to young people by a variety of agencies: co-location, out-stationing, staff loans, and joint intake and assessment. The first three of these involve the relocation of staff, either temporarily or on a longer-term basis. The fourth approach requires that two or more agencies determine the commonalties in their requests of information from clients, and find a way to collect and share this information more efficiently, while maintaining the confidentiality of client records.

1. **Co-location** involves two or more agencies having staff and facilities at the same location. This helps reduce problems clients may have in reaching a number of agencies. The close proximity of the agencies makes possible closer staff interaction and encourages cross-referrals and the formation of client-centered, integrated service procedures (such as client teams). Beyond selection of the agencies and sites for co-location, this approach may not require any additional interagency planning or coordination of services. It does provide opportunities for coordination, but the opportunities must be developed by the on-site staff.

2. **Out-stationing** refers to a situation in which staff from one agency are sent to work in the facilities of another agency. Because one agency is using another agency's facilities, coordination among the participating agencies is essential for success. Written agreements, such as memoranda of understanding, are especially important for clarifying what facilities are to be provided by the host agency and what responsibilities are to be met by the out-stationed staff persons.

3. **Staff loans** involve staff from one agency working temporarily under direct supervision of another agency on tasks assigned by that agency. This differs from outstationing since the staff is actually assigned to work for another agency. These loans may represent an interagency response to one agency's call for additional staff assistance. They are sometimes used to increase staff skill levels through exposure to new work environments. Administrators on loan from businesses can often be of great benefit to a voluntary public agency.

4. **Joint intake and assessment** can occur when agencies use a common system for screening clients and diagnosing their needs. A centralized intake point for social service providers, situated in a community setting, is one way to streamline service procedures. A client enters the system by meeting with one provider who can make referrals to other agencies as needed and who shares the initial intake form with the participating agencies after the client has provided permission to release information. This is an attempt to develop a uniform data collection system. Some agencies may find that they need only share a certain portion of their intake forms. Additional information not necessary to the purpose of other participating agencies may be collected on separate forms (Rossi, Gilmartin, and Dayton, 1986).

Development of a Coalition Information Clearinghouse

In order to improve the level of information that is shared among programs, there is a need to collect and share information collectively without threatening the confidentiality of clients. The first task is to assess what kind of information you want to collect that will be helpful to each of the participating agencies in the pregnancy prevention network.

Initially, agencies can submit their individual agency reports and tabulations to a central location where they can be organized and indexed and their availability made known to other agencies. The lead agency may choose to be designated as the central clearinghouse. The information gathered will also be important for the purpose of documenting and evaluating your coalition's efforts in adolescent pregnancy prevention. Once agencies express an interest in initiating such a clearinghouse, they should review and establish policy issues regarding confidentiality of client data and other agency data, such as specific budget expenditures.

Joint Program Design

As agencies explore the various ways in which they will collaborate and coordinate their services, they will most likely begin to explore how they can plan program operations jointly for future grant cycles. While representatives from each agency are in charge of their own program segments, monthly coalition meetings are used to assess how well the various components are operating and coordinating with one another. Management teams composed of representatives from different agencies can also work toward integrating services. Establishing these teams at both the supervisory and staff levels is also a good approach to sharing program responsibilities.

Joint Budgeting

Joint budgeting for the integrated plan may or may not be possible, depending on the funding sources. State agency or private foundation grants may stipulate that a single agency serve as the primary fiscal agent, although several agencies may be involved in the decisions affecting resource allocation. When the program operation funds are received piecemeal, with each agency supporting its own program segment, integrated budgeting may be limited to joint decision-making regarding the allocation of resources (Rossi, Gilmartin, Dayton, 1982).

The greatest potential for exploring creative approaches to sharing budgetary responsibilities lies with the administration of program resources that are generated locally in in-kind contributions, volunteer support, and private donations. Because these resources belong to the program as a whole, interagency approaches to budget administration, cost accounting, and projections of resource needs and availability can be tried. When funds for the program become a shared responsibility, standardized forms and uniform record-keeping procedures for monitoring program resources can be designed and put to use. Accounting departments within each agency should also be involved with the integration of services, particularly where budgetary constraints are concerned. It is also important to cross-reference required budget tasks and establish common procedures for all agencies involved.

Personnel

Strong leadership is essential if joint efforts are to succeed. Leaders set the tone and provide the rewards that can either encourage or squelch collaboration. Effective leadership means putting an organization's best people on the issue and giving them the authority, time and resources to do the job. It also means involving key middle- and upper-level staff members at the early stages. These line managers will later be responsible for implementation, and they will do a far better job if their input is taken seriously along the way.

Career professionals will remain in the agency long after the current political leadership has moved on. Cooperative efforts work best when the participants – individuals as well as organizations – feel that they are equal partners and consequently invest themselves fully in the endeavor. Policy changes will not be successful unless supervisors and agency managers, who will implement the changes, are engaged throughout the process.

Planners of collaborative efforts must also build interdependence among coalition participants by making sure that the staffs of one or two agencies do not control critical committees or tasks. Thus all members of the group have an investment in the success of their counterparts from other agencies.

The Media Link

The coalition can also use media at several crucial junctures in program planning and implementation. The first step in designing a media campaign is to define the specific message and the target group for whom it is intended. For example, if in your needs assessment you found that many parents of children in junior high school were unaware of the high teen pregnancy rate in your community, you might want to direct an informative message to this group.

The second step is to decide which medium will be most effective for reaching your target audience. You may want to incorporate questions in a survey of young people that asks what media channels they most often utilize. Sample questions that might be used are:

- Rank the following in terms of the time you spend on each during a typical day/ week: watching TV; listening to the radio; reading newspapers.

- What newspapers do you read? What sections?

- Which radio stations do you listen to? At what times of the day/evening?

- Which TV stations do you watch? At what times of the day/evening?

Print and broadcast media can be used to:

1. Alert the public to an issue or problem such as teen pregnancy.

2. Inform people of the presence of your program.

3. Motivate people to use program services or attend events.

Even with a limited budget you can find many affordable media sources that reach large parts of your community. For example, you could encourage a local TV or newspaper reporter who is interested in adolescent health and social issues to follow the progress of your program from the earliest stages right through planning and implementation. The different media possibilities are listed below:

Media Possibilities

- Flyers
- Posters
- News Releases
- Pamphlets and Brochures
- Paid Advertisements
- Public Service Announcements
- Comic Strips
- Question/Answer Newspaper Column

- Billboards
- Buses/Trains
- Feature Stories
- Letters to the Editor
- Editorial Page Article
- Talk Shows
- Videos for Local TV
- Teen Theater

From the results of your needs assessment you will be able to develop a report summarizing local statistics about teen pregnancy and related problems, current resources, and community awareness. Announcement of these findings can be made at a press conference that generates local media coverage.

Dissemination of the Implementation Plan

You may wish to develop an implementation plan information packet to include:

- A copy of the needs assessment findings with an explanation of the need that brought about the formation of the coalition,

- A list of coalition group members,

- A copy of the implementation plan.

Copies of support letters and resolutions in support of the plan may also be added. This packet will be particularly useful if successful implementation of the plan requires elected or appointed government bodies to take specific actions. For example, a letter of support acknowledging commitment to your plan, written by the city council, board of supervisors or others may be helpful in your efforts to gain funding.

If you are seeking specific action by government bodies in response to your strategic plan, you may need to complete the following steps in order to gain appropriate attention to your plan:

- Decide who (one or more persons) will be the most appropriate representative(s) of your coalition to contact the target body.

- Request time on a meeting agenda, ensuring that you allow enough lead time so that other group members can be present.

- Notify the media of your presentation.

- At the time of the presentation, have on hand enough copies of the implementation plan information packet for each group member you are addressing, and the press.

- Make a concise presentation of the group's findings and recommendations. Be specific as to what the group is to do.

- State that the group will follow up to determine whether and how the recommendations have been implemented.

- If the recommendation is rejected, inquire as to the reasons. Do whatever is necessary and appropriate to explore and counter these reasons. Keep trying. Through the group's actions, demonstrate that the coalition can be recognized as a credible community resource.

It is also important to designate coalition members to serve as public spokespersons for the group. They should be available to make presentations at civic and community organizations, respond to media inquiries, etc. Arrange for guest appearances on news and public affairs programs. Keep a continual flow of information to the public through news releases and letters to the editors in local papers.

Planning for Long-term Funding

It is important to consider long-term funding if you want to institute a successful plan over time. If you are successful in obtaining initial funding to develop the coalition, you most likely will be asked by the funder to provide a funding plan for future efforts in implementing the community plan on adolescent pregnancy prevention.

Most foundation sources will not be interested in maintaining your program as a long-term dependent; rather, the role of many foundations is to help initiate programs that can then be maintained by stable funding from other sources. Too often, model programs are developed without consideration of long-term funding, which may risk disillusioning both clients and the community at large. In addition to planning for future funding, it is also important to diversify the sources and kinds of funding in case any one component fails to materialize.

Ensuring future funding helps establish credibility for your project, particularly if you are seeking seed money to initiate and evaluate a program. Seed money can range from small, discretionary planning grants to larger grants that support the operational expenses of the program. Begin to line up some of this planned commitment as a way of demonstrating support and broad community involvement. Having the commitment of funding partners (several sources of funding collaborating to support the project) on paper through a memorandum of agreement or letter of support will greatly enhance your additional fundraising efforts.

Here are some suggestions for ways in which funding for model programs can be continued on an ongoing basis:

1. If the organization is large enough, the program's success will require managers to examine how the current budget can be reallocated to support this new effort. This is perhaps more acceptable within an organization when the new effort already builds upon current activities of the organization. For example, if the new component is coordination of services aimed at enhancing community outreach and decreasing overlapping efforts by parallel agencies, the organization may soon learn that a coordinator position is important to improve organizational efficiency. Demonstrating that your program has assumed funding responsibilities for successful pilot projects in the past is one of the strongest arguments for your ability to do it in the future. In addition, it is important to delineate what "in-kind" contributions your organization is already providing as a partnership in initiating this new effort. The specific value of the "in-kind" support, including administrative support, should be included as part of the proposed budget.

2. If your program has a "fee-for-service" potential (to be financed by the clients, perhaps on a sliding scale, or most likely by a third-party payor), then document the potential client population, including what you know about their income level, fees paid for comparable services, and evidence of the clients' ability to pay some fees in order to obtain reimbursement for services. Based on the profile of the clients you are most likely to serve, you can begin to project an anticipated income that will develop over the life of the project. However, in considering this source of income it is important to take into account start-up time. This will most likely mean planning for fewer clients at the beginning of the project, and for seasonal variations, such as those related to school schedules and vacations.

   Be sure to identify the potential payors with whom you might contract to provide care and services. Assess whether the coalition or the individual agencies within the coalition qualify to be contractors. Developing such contractual relationships takes time, including the time necessary to develop a mechanism for billing and completing reimbursement paperwork. If the program effort appears promising, plan to include in your second year budget a sufficient proportion of the coordinator's time (or that of a special consultant) to develop these reimbursement mechanisms.

   In a few school-based health centers, adolescents are charged an annual fee of $25 per person to use the program. A sliding scale is also established in order to prevent adolescents from experiencing a barrier to care. These fees, while comprising only a small part of the overall budget, contribute to the functioning of the program and demonstrate to funders the involvement of the target population. Furthermore, staff feel it is important that adolescents learn about the necessity of paying for a medical service.

3. The coalition or participating members might be able to develop a non-grant fundraising program to support parts of the plan. Community-based organizations often sponsor raffles, auctions and fund drives to raise a portion of their overall budget. If your organization is already involved in a yearly fundraising effort of this type, then you will need to consider whether this effort can be expanded. Based on past history, you can project how much money might be raised and whether it will be worth the time and investment. Often members of the advisory board or volunteers can carry many of these responsibilities. You will most likely have to develop a "contingency" plan in case these fundraising efforts are not successful. Also, explore what funding channels are possible through community fundraising efforts, such as United Way, and what is required in order to qualify for these sources of revenue and be part of their budget allocation.

4. The coalition or individual programs may have a profitable service or activity that can be expanded to cover the costs of sponsoring the new program effort. Perhaps

your organization is already selling publications, or providing consulting services to other groups, and can generate the funding necessary to cover expenses of implementing the coalition's strategic plan. If this is one avenue for revenue, you must plan what kind of expansion will be necessary to support the expanded service program.

5. Organizations within the coalition might be in a position to assume financial and program responsibility for implementing the coalition's plan. For example, if some of the life options strategies appear to increase the numbers of students who successfully graduate from high school, the schools might incorporate the program into their budget (particularly if there is an increase in attendance, which contributes to the overall income of the school). As another example, local employers might sponsor a number of students receiving a special training program begun at the high school level, particularly if this work force is ready to begin work right after graduation.

Potential Sources of Funding

A number of private and public funding sources may be available to your community in its efforts to implement the community-wide plan. Gathering information about which foundations are committed to youth development issues in general, and specifically to adolescent pregnancy prevention, is an important first step.

The Foundation Center, funded by private foundations, assists potential applicants in identifying appropriate foundations for particular proposals. It publishes a variety of helpful materials available for purchase and in libraries. Among these materials is the Foundation Directory, which provides information on the nation's largest foundations – those with assets of $1 million or more, or that make annual grants of at least $1,000. The directory has a geographical index, an index divided into types of support (endowments, capital support, seed money) and a subject index. Each index indicates which foundations give grants on a national basis and which limit their giving to the state or city in which they are located.

You can also obtain this information through an on-line computer search. "Comsearch Printouts" can also be purchased from the Foundation Center. These printouts list foundation grants of over $5,000 in specific topic areas, such as health. The grants are grouped geographically. The main office of the Foundation Center also maintains microfiche of foundations' tax records, thus enabling you to find out who their current grantees are and the kinds and amounts of grants awarded. (You can get the same information yourself from the individual foundations by writing to request an annual report.) The Foundation Center also maintains a collection of books published by others that list foundation giving by state. Their main office in New York will help you identify the library in your area that houses Foundation Center resources. Your local library may contain Foundation Center materials as well as other materials on local foundations.

Private Sources

Local foundations often support demonstration projects, particularly in their initial phase of development. This support in turn helps to attract other state or national funding. Small local foundations often assist in advocating for the programs they fund and in finding additional sources of revenue. They may provide a matching grant, in which the agency raises funds that are in turn matched dollar for dollar by the foundation. Local foundations may maintain a long commitment to the project once it is developed.

National foundations are often attracted to the broad topic of youth development issues, rather than specifically adolescent pregnancy, although a number of foundations are fully committed to this particular problem area. National foundations tend to fund grants that support either a new model approach or a program innovation.

Traditionally, foundation grants are devoted to the initial phase of a program's operation and are rarely used for ongoing service delivery. However, since your community-wide program will most likely be implemented in phases as the community gains experience in providing integrated services, different foundations may be interested in providing funding for different components or stages. Foundations generally prefer not to be the sole provider of a program's funding base, so they will prefer to find that you have alternative long-term funding strategies. National foundations may also be interested in developing matching funding collaborations with public funders. Such a successful experiment has been the combining of funding from the "Ounce of Prevention Fund" and the Illinois Department of Human Services.

Public Sources

Public monies are essential to maintaining the funding of your project, particularly as most private foundations consider their major contribution to the field is in developing innovative programs. It is best to secure public sector funding as soon as possible, and it is likely that your current collaborative partners are already involved in receiving some public funding. The funding sources highlighted in Chapter 3 may be helpful to you. They include at the federal level, the Maternal and Child Health (MCH) Block Grant (Title V) of the Public Health Services Act, which provides services for youth as part of its maternal and child health programs, including comprehensive preventive care services with case management and follow-up care; Section 330 Community Based Health Centers, which provide care in medically underserved communities; Medicaid, the primary source of health care coverage for the poor; and Early Periodic Screening, Diagnostic and Treatment Services (EPSDT), one of several Medicaid programs providing assistance.

At the state level, two types of major funds exist: monies generated by the state through taxes and other revenue sources, and monies from federal block grants, which the state allocates in accordance with its own priorities and rules. The use of state resources for innovative programs may require "demonstration" grants or general funding authorization, as well as allocations of monies through a regular budget process. Typically, these are line items attached to the health department's appropriation and budget. Other state generated funds may be available for a broad range of youth-related programs that do not require a specified line item or authorization (Hadley, Lovick, and Kirby, 1986).

Funding from city or county sources is another possibility. Many cities are beginning to explore strategies for addressing such problems as teenage pregnancy and may be interested in supporting broad-based community projects. State substance abuse programs, juvenile justice programs, job training, and employment projects may all be tapped to help.

Locating Public Funding Sources

You may begin the process of locating potential public funding sources by identifying communities that have implemented similar projects and documenting their sources of funding. People working in these community-based programs will most often be generous in sharing this information with you. Other individuals who will be helpful are staff members in state agencies who are familiar with the types of funding sources that exist at both the state and federal levels. Individuals working in the field of youth development within your community will also be helpful in identifying potential sources of funding. For example, if you have a job training component in your community-wide strategy, you should begin with agencies that are already receiving funding in this arena. It will be of even greater benefit if these individual agencies are part of your coalition and are active allies. Their current funding may be relevant to your project, particularly if it can leverage existing funds. These agencies may also be most knowledgeable about funding trends in their specific fields and what kind of match may exist between your community plan and the priorities of funding agencies (Hadley, Lovick, and Kirby, 1986).

Other individuals who may be able to help you are members of the state legislature, and staff members of relevant legislative committees. They may be particularly helpful to you in identifying the individual within the funding agency whom it will be most useful to contact. Often a letter of support from legislators will greatly facilitate your entry.

In-kind Services

In-kind contributions are an important part of any community-based effort. They can often cover the full costs of a service or staff member, or can be used in concert with other funding. For instance you may hire a half-time social worker, one-quarter of whose time might be an in-kind donation (supported by another program) and the other quarter contracted through the overall coalition.

There are several types of in-kind services:

• Space, including maintenance and utilities for that space,

- Professional staffing, including counselors and school nurses donated by the school district,

- Health professionals in training,

- Clerical assistance,

- Services (e.g. laboratory and diagnostic services from the health department),

- Equipment and furniture,

- Construction and renovation,

- Printing facilities,

- Transportation,

- Public relations and promotional activities,

- Recreational activities.

Assess what other youth-serving agencies, local departments of health, social service organizations and school administrators are contributing (or could expand) in terms of in-kind support. This can be crucial in implementing the plan. (See Appendix 7-2 for a worksheet on what each agency needs and can provide.)

Developing a Budget

Developing a budget, particularly one that overlaps a number of agencies participating in the coalition, will require extensive coordination. Unless the coalition becomes a formal, incorporated entity, it is likely that the lead agency will be responsible for submitting a proposal and accompanying budget. Though the work will be conducted by numerous agencies, one fiscal agency must maintain accountability for the operating budget. Most lead agencies will have facilities for monitoring the budget.

Depending upon the level of responsibility of the participating agencies, subcontracts among the major partners will most likely be necessary. Some funding agencies will only pay one set of overhead costs; thus alternative payment systems may have to be considered — for example, paying part of the salary of another agency's staff member directly, or placing that person in the budget of the lead agency. Most agencies have restrictions on the percentage of time an employee must be employed in order to qualify for insurance and other benefits. Thus, it is important to coordinate with the staff's primary employer how salaries and benefits will be handled. In addition, many foundations will not pay administrative overhead.

Though you will not know all the specific costs of the proposed program, the budget provides your most educated estimate of what it takes to accomplish your goals. Once you have begun the project, you may need to modify and revise within the allocated funding to accommodate unexpected changes.

Most budgets are comprised of two major components: personnel costs and non-personnel costs. Within each component, it is important to delineate what funding is being formally requested and what funding is already being contributed, as well as your total costs. Under personnel costs, identify specific staff who will be working on the project, their salaries, amount of time, and level of effort. Fringe benefits should be included as a separate category. Some of the organizations in your coalition may require that you state salary ranges for each position (Kiritz, 1980).

Under personnel costs, most budgets have a separate item for consulting services, which may include the costs of the evaluation component and other efforts by coalition members. Both paid and volunteer consultants would be listed in this section; donated salaries should reflect normal salaries or consulting fees.

Non-personnel costs include office space, utilities, maintenance, janitorial services, and rental, lease, or purchase of equipment. Other supply costs include desk-top supplies and copying expenses. Travel is another important component, and depending upon how much driving you anticipate as part of the implementation plan, project the number of miles you expect each person to drive each month. Multiply the number of miles by the acceptable reimbursement rate in local agencies, and by the number of months in the grant period. (For example: Local Mileage for Project Coordinator — 100 miles a month at 23 cents per mile x 12 months). You may also project the costs of attending a program-related meeting or training. These items should be supported by a statement in your budget justification that describes the benefits of attending the meeting.

Indirect costs or overhead costs cover a percentage of expenses incurred in sponsoring a project. Indirect costs may or may not be provided by any particular funding sources. Some funding sources place a ceiling upon indirect costs in specific situations. Sometimes indirect costs are a percentage of the total direct costs or of the personnel costs, or of the salary and wages items alone.

Proposal Writing

Contact each foundation or other funding source and obtain guidelines for submitting a proposal. Follow these guidelines precisely. Some funding sources will simply ask you to submit your proposal, your budget, and information about your organization. Others will ask you to write an introductory letter, briefly outlining your proposal. From this summary, they will decide whether you should submit a formal proposal. Always keep an eye on deadlines; set up a timeline and stick to it.

The style of the proposal is up to you, but how you pitch the program may determine whether or not you get the grant. Your proposal needs to be in tune with the foundation's objectives. Some grant seekers write a master proposal that elaborates on all topics of probable interest to funders; they then adjust the proposal's content and form in accordance with particular foundation requirements.

Do not make the mistake of changing your activities to fit the goals of a certain funder. Apply for funds only when appropriate. When you decide to submit a proposal, make certain the language you use to describe your planned programs relates to the funder's objectives. For example, if a foundation is interested in youth self-sufficiency it would be useful to outline the ways your program components relate to this objective (Hadley, Lovick, and Kirby, 1986).

Key Proposal
Ingredients

1. General outline – an overall brief summary of your proposal.

2. Objective or goal – a brief statement about what you hope to accomplish with the grant.

3. Problem – a short overview or description of the nature of the problem you hope to address. If adolescent health is the focus, then summarize the status of adolescent health in your community.

4. Need – describe the need that you hope to address, based upon the results of the needs assessment.

5. Program Plan – a description of what you propose to do and a definition of how each activity relates to need. Program plans should also include a description of the coalition and the following:

   a. Proposed services

   b. Program's relationship to school

   c. Program's relationship to parents

   d. Program's relationship to the community

6. Other funding sources – an indication of your plans for other funding.

7. Organizational capacity – an explanation of why your group is qualified to undertake this program. Describe the experience and expertise you have that demonstrates your ability to carry out this endeavor.

8. Budget – an outline of your specific budget

Obtaining funding will be an ongoing process for the coalition, and it is likely that each year you will need to pursue new funding possibilities. An ongoing fund development committee should be actively pursuing funding options and developing alternative fundraising strategies.

Be Prepared to Revise the Implementation Plan

The implementation plan should include feedback mechanisms to enable the coalition to periodically take stock of what is being accomplished and to make revisions in the plan as data suggest. As the plan enters a second year of effort, it will be especially important to have this feedback. If different agencies are accountable for sections of the plan, the coalition will need to monitor their performance and identify where additional assistance, resources, and revised expectations may be necessary.

Continue to hold meetings of the coalition to review progress, barriers, successes, and failures on each component of the program. Reassess goals, objectives and procedures periodically, based on feedback and evaluation. Be flexible. Submit the modified plan to collaborating agencies as appropriate. Continue to monitor implementation, and repeat the process if necessary to reach the desired goal.

Summary

Many months (perhaps years) of preliminary work by coalition members lead them to the point of implementing their community strategies. Inevitably, the two most basic issues the coalition must deal with become:

1. How to maintain a coalition that will facilitate the kind of interagency coordination necessary to implement the group's plan, and

2. How to maintain a stable funding base in order to carry out the objectives of the coalition.

The discussion in this chapter has focused on these factors – the strength of the coalition and long-term funding – because they are fundamental to the group's ultimate success. Once the implementation phase of the plan has begun, the coalition now produces a viable, living, changing program that requires close monitoring and study, as well as reassessment and revision, in order to ensure its survival as an effective community organization. This leads us to the next and final chapter in our guide – a discussion of evaluation and its key role in the coalition's activities.

Appendix 7-1

Force Field Analysis

*A*useful strategy is the incorporation of a force field analysis, originally developed by Dr. Kurt Lewin, which helps identify conditions that support attainment of a goal and those that block its attainment. The use of Force Field Analysis can be an effective approach to building group consensus and to developing effective strategies for resolving a community's problems (Kitzi, 1987). It can help a coalition determine what strategies to include in the community-wide plan. Once several strategies have been prioritized, the committee can brainstorm all the alternative solutions toward implementing these options. Based on the results of Force Field Analysis, an implementation plan can be created that includes your goals and measurable objectives.

List under each of the selected goals all the behaviors or actions required to reach that goal. Consider who else you should include to work on these steps, where, how, and when to start. Establish a time frame, with tasks listed in chronological order. It is important that you record the action plan, and document who will be responsible for implementing its components. Recognize that plans may be changed as data about implementation of the plan are collected. At every juncture, however, agreements and responsibilities should be clearly understood, and any changes negotiated with all members of the coalition.

The problem in this case is the gap between what exists and what is desired. The conditions that preclude reaching the goal are called "blocking forces". The "supporting forces" are the positive factors which move the group closer toward the goal. The following steps for conducting a force field analysis are applied to one possible adolescent pregnancy prevention goal — increasing the numbers of students who earn their high school diplomas without experiencing an unintended pregnancy.

1. Clearly state the specific goal that you want to accomplish, as well as the situation that currently exists.

2. Using brainstorming techniques, list all the factors currently in place that should help you reach the goal (+ factors). These are driving forces towards the goal. For example:

   a. Renewed interest in improving educational experiences for young people

   b. Strong commitment by parents and other family members to attaining higher education

   c. State regulations regarding school enrollment for minors

   d. Availability of special partnerships between businesses and schools committed to having students continue with their education.

3. In the same way, list the forces which prevent you from changing the situation (– factors) and which might stand in the way of accomplishing your goal. For example:

   a. Lack of good jobs for young people with only a high school diploma, which discourages many youngsters from completing their requirements

   b. Lack of viable role models who have successfully completed their education

   c. Enticements of drug-selling world, where kids can make a substantial amount of money

   d. Schools that appear to push out hard-to-teach students

Example:

Current Situation:
High Adolescent Pregnancy Rate Related to High School Dropout Rate

+	**—**	**GOAL**
• Interest in improving education	• Lack of viable jobs with HS diploma	Increase numbers of adolescents who complete school and delay childbearing
• Strong commitment by parents	• Lack of viable role models	
• State regulations re: school enrollment	• Enticements of drug-selling world	
• Business/school partnerships	• Schools push out the hard-to-teach	

4. When all the driving (+) and restraining (–) forces have been listed, you will need to decide on the strength of each force. How big or how important are the forces in relation to reaching or blocking your goal? You will note that the co-existing counterpressures help to maintain the current situation as you encounter it today in your community.

5. After listing all the forces you can think of, you should:

a. Rank each factor in terms of its degree of significance. Thus, a #1 would represent a factor that is vitally important in either positively or negatively influencing the achievement of the goal. Rank each of the factors that has been proposed so that each factor has a numerical value.

b. Next, rate each factor 1, 2, or 3 to reflect the difficulty or ease of changing that factor, with a 3 representing a very difficult factor to change, a 2 representing a medium difficulty in changing the force, and a 1 representing a factor that is easy to change.

Thus, you may find that while changing the number one restraining factor would have the greatest impact, the difficulty of changing it would be so challenging as to defeat your efforts. You may opt to work on a factor of lesser importance, but one that is easier to change. Beginning with greater odds for success improves your chances of building community confidence in your efforts.

The following action choices are available for the coalition to consider in developing an action plan:

a. Diminish the strongest negative force or forces. Choose those that you can do something about, and brainstorm all the things you could do to weaken or eliminate their strength.

b. Strengthen the strongest positives. Brainstorm all the things that you could do to strengthen these forces.

c. Combine strong positives, if possible. For example, are there various resources that you could combine to expand current efforts directed towards preventing school dropout?

d. Work toward reversing a strong negative into a strong positive.

e. Remove negative forces, if possible.

The most likely option is to diminish the strongest "doable" negative force and use it as a basis for developing an incremental approach to achieving your objectives.

Appendix 7-2

What You Can Gain or Provide Through Interagency Coordination

Worksheet 7-2	Your Agency Needs	Your Agency Has to Offer
Staff		
■ Professional expertise on certain topics	☐	☐
■ Staff with interests in certain types of clients	☐	☐
■ Staff with particular skills (statistical, writing, counseling, testing, interviewing)	☐	☐
■ Secretarial or clerical help	☐	☐
■ Other	☐	☐
Equipment		
■ Typing	☐	☐
■ Duplication	☐	☐
■ Word processing	☐	☐
■ Computer	☐	☐
■ Media-related (audiovisual)	☐	☐
■ Other	☐	☐
Facilities		
■ Office space	☐	☐
■ Conference room	☐	☐
■ Counseling rooms	☐	☐
■ Office furniture	☐	☐
■ Advantageous location	☐	☐
■ Other	☐	☐
Information		
■ On client needs	☐	☐

- On community needs   ☐   ☐
- Other   ☐   ☐

Services
- Informational   ☐   ☐
- Testing   ☐   ☐
- Counseling   ☐   ☐
- Treatment   ☐   ☐
- Placement   ☐   ☐
- Other   ☐   ☐

Contacts
- With current and potential clients   ☐   ☐
- With employers   ☐   ☐
- With other agencies   ☐   ☐
- With funding sources   ☐   ☐
- With community leaders   ☐   ☐
- With state or federal officials   ☐   ☐
- Other   ☐   ☐

Chapter 8

Evaluating the
Community-wide Plan

E valuation is a process for determining the value of a program. The findings of an evaluation allow planners and funding agencies to assess what is working and what is not; to determine what factors contribute to the success or failure of the program; and to ascertain how well the needs of the target population are being met. It is then possible to make decisions concerning what components of the effort to maintain, and what to change. Evaluation results are compared with:

1. Anticipated outcomes as established by original objectives of the coalition, and

2. Standards established in the field of community pregnancy prevention interventions.

The results allow funding agencies to estimate the value of future funding. Evaluation results can also be used to improve and gain support for additional teen pregnancy prevention effort.

Planning the evaluation should occur concurrently with the design of the project. Beginning an evaluation after implementation of a program can seriously limit available options for collecting information. In order to collect baseline information from participants, sources and mechanisms for data collection must be established early on.

Why evaluate?

• To monitor the progress of a program,

• To determine the impact of an effort on the community,

- To determine whether each program component is meeting its objectives in an effective manner,

- To communicate with the community about the contributions of the interventions,

- To aid in making funding decisions, including how best to allocate human and fiscal resources,

- To improve a program's activities and services,

- To meet the requirements of funding agencies,

- To establish the need for and value of additional funding.

The needs assessment can serve as baseline documentation of how the community is functioning before implementation of the program. The evaluation must be designed to monitor the effects of each component as well as the total, since different strategies will be added on an incremental basis and may well be aimed at addressing an assortment of issues. Given that a combination of strategies and services will be implemented, it is imperative that the evaluation help ascertain which programs contribute to expected outcomes for the target population.

Types of Evaluation

Four primary types of evaluation have been developed to examine different components in program development:

- Process

- Outcome

- Impact

- Effectiveness

1. **Process** evaluation looks at the way a program has conformed to its design, and the extent to which it is producing all the materials and services promised. Process evaluation can also examine any barriers that might prevent achievement of the objectives, and identify ways to overcome these factors. Here are some questions of relevance:

   - Are appropriate personnel, equipment and financial resources available in the right quantity, in the right place, and at the right time to meet program needs? If not, what barriers are preventing these activities from taking place?

- Are expected "products" of the program actually being provided? Is the program providing the expected services, and reaching the target population?

- What key ingredients contribute to the results being achieved?

- Are the activities being completed on time? Is the time-line adequate to reach the established objectives?

Case Example
_____

A community-based teen pregnancy prevention project planned a five-pronged approach based on findings from the needs assessment. The five components included: 1) comprehensive family life education in the schools, 2) communication skills workshops for teens and their parents, 3) special teen hours at the local family planning clinic, 4) enhancing the referral system from the school and social service agencies to the teen family planning clinic, and 5) a media campaign informing the community of the high teen pregnancy rate and of the facilities available to prevent it. The first component of the community's evaluation plan was a process evaluation to determine if the program components were in place after the designated time-line and, if not, to assess what barriers were blocking this implementation. The evaluation showed that the first three components were operating, although the family life education had been delayed by two months due to an extended review of materials by the school board. The fourth component, enhancing referral to the teen clinic, had met some obstacles as well. An essential activity, training of health and social service workers, had been held up due to the reluctance of department heads to add additional activities to their staffs' responsibilities. The fifth objective, the media campaign, was put on hold because of a shortage of people available to implement it. A revised time-line was developed as a result of the process evaluation, including closer monitoring of progress on components of the community plan.

2. **Outcome** evaluations determine whether the program has met the stated objectives. Emphasis is placed on the immediate results of program efforts. Relevant questions are:

   - Did the program meet its stated objectives? For example, did teenagers enrolled in a five-part family life education program increase knowledge of contraceptive methods by the projected 25 percent?

   - What were the short-term results of the interventions?

   - Can the results of the program be attributed to the program itself (as opposed to other factors and influences)?

Case Example *The objective of an advertising campaign was to increase membership in an after-school teen center by 30 percent within a six-month period. The planning committee had agreed to try school announcements and flyers. Program managers documented how many teens were enrolled, and monitored the number of new teenagers participating after the initial information campaign. After two months, there was only a 10 percent increase. In order to increase enrollment, radio announcements and special contests held at the center were added. The evaluation documented that with these outreach efforts, participation increased by 35 percent, with the majority of new members reporting that they found out about the center through the media campaign. Program managers also documented process measures such as the number of flyers distributed, radio announcements made, and the teens' response to the different center activities.*

3. **Impact** evaluations determine whether the program ultimately had the desired long-term effect. Measures are more related to achievement of goals than are outcome evaluations. Questions central to this type of evaluation are:

    • Did a particular program produce the desired effect? For example, did it reduce the rate of unintended pregnancy?

    • Could the observed effects have occurred in the absence of the program, or in the presence of some alternative program?

Case Example *A youth-serving agency wanted to address the problem of large numbers of teens dropping out of school, and a subsequent high unemployment rate as a result of unintended pregnancy. Agency planners selected a comprehensive approach with a strong emphasis on life-options strategies. Their program included a school re-entry program for pregnant and parenting teenagers, support groups for teens, school-work placements that paid students stipends, a job training program, listings of job openings for teens, family life education, and referrals to the family planning clinic. Measures of the impact of this program included rates of school continuation and employment, and numbers of teen births, which were compared for five years before and after the program was implemented, and compared to a similar community without a comprehensive plan.*

4. **Efficiency** evaluations determine if program results are being obtained in the most cost-efficient manner. Pertinent questions are:

    • Does the program show enough effects given the costs?

    • Are program benefits more or less expensive per unit of outcome than benefits from other programs designed to achieve the same goal?

Case Example

A family planning clinic was interested in extending the amount of time spent at intake, and the amount of interpersonal skills counseling made available to their teen clients. To determine if the additional costs associated with increased time with clients would results in better contraceptive compliance and fewer pregnancies, the clinic assigned half its clients to the new counseling approach and half to the traditional counseling services for six months. The evaluation showed that increased counseling time was more expensive, but was cost-effective, in that contraceptive compliance was increased, particularly for those at highest risk of pregnancy. The evaluation also helped develop a profile of teens who were at highest risk of being clinic dropouts. As a result, the clinic developed a "triage" system and began using the new counseling approach for high-risk teens.

Since each type of evaluation will answer different questions, you will want to choose a combination of approaches. For example, suppose you use an impact measure such as teen pregnancy rates. Because many factors affect the pregnancy rate, it might be very difficult to document that your intervention was solely or primarily responsible for an observed change. So in addition to this impact measure, you will also want to collect process and outcome data on individual components of your intervention. For example, in looking at the effectiveness of your health education efforts, you may document the increase in knowledge among program participants, the number of participants enrolled, the intent to avoid pregnancies among participants and nonparticipants, and reports by participants on improvements in parent-child communication.

If your program was able to demonstrate positive outcomes, you will want to know:

- What mediating factors contributed to its success?

- What components were the most effective?

- How can you continue to improve the program?

- What problems remain?

In addition to helping to improve your program, this information will allow for its potential replication in other communities.

What Should You Evaluate?

Decisions concerning the extent of the evaluation will depend upon:

1. The objectives of your programs and the community-wide effort

2. The questions you want to answer; and

3. The financial and human resources available.

Included in your program plan will be objectives describing programmatic inputs (process objectives), short-term effects of your programs (outcome objectives), and long-term effects of your community-wide effort (impact objectives). The differences among these objectives are described in detail later in this chapter.

Process Objectives

In order to satisfy the demands of the funding agency and to allow the coordinator to function effectively you will need to be able to determine if your program's process objectives have been met. An accurate record-keeping system allows you to track the progress of a program or combination of programs and to answer critical process questions, giving the program manager or community-wide coordinator the information they need to make decisions concerning distribution of resources. Here are examples of questions to ask when process objectives are assessed:

- Has the adolescent community services network been established according to plan?

- Has the family life education program reached 1,000 adolescents, as intended?

- Are out-of-school youths utilizing the teen center?

Outcome Objectives

Another set of questions concerns the short-term outcomes. Did teens learn how to say "no" to unwanted sex? Did those who are sexually active learn how to obtain and use contraceptives? Did parents participating in communications classes report talking to their teens more often? If you wrote outcome objectives into your plan, then your evaluation plan must allow you to assess whether these objectives have been attained.

Impact Objectives

The third type of question concerns the impact of your entire community-based effort. Did the teen pregnancy rate decrease? Did the high school dropout rate go down? In order to assess changes in these areas, you will need to put a great deal of effort, and significant resources, into an evaluation plan; and this will most likely require the assistance of evaluation experts as well as use of a control or comparison group.

The cost of conducting the evaluation usually increases as you move from process to outcome and to impact evaluations. Each phase of this evaluation spectrum requires more time and expertise in order to obtain an accurate picture of your efforts. A poorly planned and poorly conducted evaluation may likely present incomplete, inaccurate and inadequate findings. For a variety of reasons, including a weakening of the original program intervention, quality of data collected, and lack of access to an equivalent comparison group, even the most carefully planned evaluation effort may not be able to demonstrate a statistically significant impact of a program.

There is often a temptation to collect as much information as possible, rather than collecting only the information that is really needed to conduct the evaluation. It is important not to overburden staff, program resources, and participants with excessive information that could well compromise the quality of the data collected.

A major factor in deciding how extensive your evaluation will be is what you want to learn from your efforts. If you are considering replicating your program in other communities you will need to demonstrate that the community-wide effort did, in fact, have an impact on the targeted community.

Examples

Decision Analysis

To make the best use of your evaluation results, the first task is to identify the questions that are important for future decisions. Identifying information needed to support or reject plans allows evaluation results to be directly linked to decision making.

Step 1: Identify the decisions that will be based on the evaluation results. Consider all stakeholders when identifying potential decisions.

> *Example: Whether to expand the number and type of agencies participating in the Adolescent Health Services Network.*

Step 2: Identify what criteria you will use to make this decision.

> *Example: Was coordination among participating agencies enhanced? Was duplication or overlapping of services decreased and comprehensiveness increased?*

Step 3: Identify the information that will be needed from the evaluation to answer these questions.

> *Example: Information concerning how coordination efforts have affected comprehensiveness of assistance received by youths.*
> *Information concerning the cost-effectiveness of a coordinated array of services.*

(Adapted from Agencies Working Together by Rossi, Gilmartin and Dayton, Sage Human Services Guide 28, 1982.)

Who Should Evaluate?

To decide who will lead the evaluation effort, and to consider related questions, an evaluation subcommittee of the coalition should be formed. It is particularly helpful to include people from the coalition as well as others in the community who have had experience conducting evaluations. If you are able to identify individuals within the coalition who have evaluation skills, you may decide to do an internal evaluation. If the pool of skills does not include evaluation, it is highly advisable to obtain technical assistance from an outside evaluator, such as one from either a university or private consulting firm. You may need help to design and implement evaluation strategies and to assist in the data analysis, or you may want all evaluations to be done by outsiders. In many respects, an evaluation conducted from outside will increase the credibility of the evaluation efforts and will help guard against internal biases or program pressures to show the "right" results. Universities, particularly departments of psychology, sociology, public health and education, can usually identify professionals with the necessary skills.

One role of your evaluation subcommittee may be to seek additional funding for the evaluation component, since not all funding sources are interested in paying for a comprehensive evaluation. However, there is increasing interest in being able to determine "what works", and many foundations and public agencies will even require that an evaluation component be in place before they are willing to fund the overall program.

Planning an Evaluation

The evaluation plan should be the result of decisions based on:

• Financial and personnel resources available to conduct the evaluation

• The goals and objectives of the community-wide plan

• The specific program components and activities designed to achieve the objectives

• Requirements of funding sources

• Expected use of the evaluation findings

• Characteristics of the target population

• Experience and skills in evaluation

The evaluation plan will specify who will do what, when, how often, and in what manner. A great deal of time and effort goes into making these procedural decisions, and you may find that as the program and the evaluation evolve, changes in the evaluation plan will be necessary. Decisions will be based on the decision-maker's knowledge of the program and the community it serves. At each step, the evaluator must communicate with staff regarding the purpose and utility of the program evaluation component. Staff members can be instrumental in providing feedback on evaluation instruments and protocols, and must be involved in establishing how and when data will be collected. Their cooperation and active participation are of paramount importance in facilitating data collection. One must also recognize that conducting an evaluation can be a major expense for a program, in personnel costs, computer costs, data analysis, and report writing.

Below is an example of an evaluation management plan covering activities for one component of a program for each week of a three-month period. It is important to gain input and feedback from as many staff members as possible on the proposed evaluation plan. Establish realistic expectations of how much time each activity will take, especially if there are competing demands. The sample worksheet will help you develop your own evaluation management plan.

Example

Sample Evaluation Management Plan

Activity	Person Responsible	Person Days	March	April	May	...
1. Review needs assessment and last year's evaluation findings for planning the program	Project Dir	1	■			
2. Revise program if necessary	Project Dir / Health Edctr	2 / 5	■			
3. Determine this year's data collection methods	Project Dir / Health Edctr	3 / 3	■			
4. Develop draft of new instrument	Health Edctr / Admn Asst	5 / 1		■		
5. Pilot test new draft	Health Edctr	3		■		
6. Make any necessary revisions	Health Edctr / Admn Asst	2 / 1			■	
7. Administer new instrument along with program	Health Edctr	10			■	

Evaluation Manual

In order to produce confidence in the findings of the evaluation, follow procedural measures consistently. A manual documenting the procedures to be followed in conducting the evaluation will contribute toward maintaining consistency. When changes are made in the protocol, they should be documented. If the original decision-maker leaves the program, a mechanism is needed for continuing with the evaluation; a new evaluator should not have to remake the decisions and cannot recreate the conditions under which they were made.

The evaluation manual, like an employee or clinic procedure manual, should specify what procedures should be followed, how, when, and why. As you are planning the evaluation, begin to construct this evaluation manual. Write down specific notes as to what is to be done and why it was decided to do things that way. This information will also be helpful when you analyze results. For example, if you decided to target a certain population, you should document how you chose that group.

Much of the process of evaluation is evolutionary in nature. As lessons are learned about your specific program evaluation, they can be applied to future evaluation efforts. Evaluation is a dynamic process. Your manual will assist you in clarifying the purpose of the evaluation and will help you collect data on a more consistent basis.

Steps In The Evaluation Process

As you begin your evaluation, consider the specific steps that will be necessary to successfully complete the evaluation. Although the process is presented in the diagram below as a step-by-step progression, remember that some steps may occur concurrently, while others must be taken sequentially. Be flexible and be prepared to modify your plan when appropriate. These steps can be utilized as the backbone of your evaluation manual.

Steps In The Evaluation Planning Process

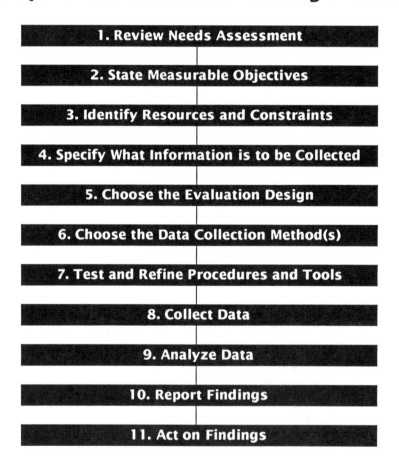

1. Review Needs Assessment
2. State Measurable Objectives
3. Identify Resources and Constraints
4. Specify What Information is to be Collected
5. Choose the Evaluation Design
6. Choose the Data Collection Method(s)
7. Test and Refine Procedures and Tools
8. Collect Data
9. Analyze Data
10. Report Findings
11. Act on Findings

Step 1: Review Needs Assessment

Describing the target population and assessing its needs is the first step in the implementation of any program. It allows you to more narrowly define the problem and the group in need of services. For example, you may learn that the age group in the community that is experiencing the greatest life-long impact of pregnancy is 17 years and below. Traditional efforts at reaching this population through family life education programs have not been successful. In addition, many adolescents leave school before family life education is provided. As a result of your needs assessment, your community-wide strategies will focus on addressing issues of life options, providing health care services, and improving self-esteem and decision-making skills. The needs assessment creates an overall baseline against which subsequent change can be measured.

Step 2: State Measurable Objectives

Objectives are specific indicators of your program's goals. They must be measurable so that you can determine to what extent they have been met. The objectives you wrote when developing your community-wide plan, which reflect the needs assessment findings, are used to establish the evaluation specifications. They are the guidelines that determine what direction the evaluation should take. Establishing realistic and specific objectives is crucial to your evaluation process.

Formula for Stating Objectives

1. Use a strong active verb (e.g. increase, start, identify).

2. State only one purpose or aim with each objective.

3. Specify a single result or end product.

4. Specify the expected time frame for achievement.

For example:

- Students will demonstrate a 20% increase in knowledge from baseline to post-test measurement after completing a three-week family life education curriculum.

- A comprehensive drop-in youth center which provides case management services will reduce the school drop-out rate by 10% in two years.

An extensive array of community strategies may be adopted as part of the community-wide plan, and it is highly unlikely that all of these can be evaluated. Not every program will have process, outcome, and impact objectives. For example, you may not be able to determine the effects of a media campaign, although you will certainly want to document that all program components were in place. Although many communities will not have the means to conduct a thorough impact evaluation, almost all will need to document what *did* occur. Whether the community is establishing brand new programs or trying to make the current roster of programs function more effectively, the total number of clients served also needs to be documented. In the communities aiming to improve existing services, the documentation might demonstrate that while the overall number of adolescents served did not change, they were reached with a much more comprehensive array of services.

Communities may also choose to evaluate discrete program components at different times, while maintaining overall program documentation. For example, evaluating the process and outcome objectives of a family life education program may be the focus of the first two years of the evaluation, while the school remediation and/or job apprenticeship programs may be evaluated during the second and third year of the programs, after the pilot plan of these projects has been completed.

Finally, the community may decide to focus its outcome and impact evaluation at the individual, service system, and policy levels. For example, outcomes such as knowledge, attitude, and behavior change resulting from exposure to the program interventions can be assessed for each individual. In addition, service system changes, such as increases in the type and comprehensiveness of services being offered, can be evaluated; so can policy changes, such as school board adoption of a mandated comprehensive family life education program.

In the example opposite, you will notice some overlap in impact objectives between individual programs and the community-wide effort: they both seek to reduce the birth rate to teens and the number of high school dropouts. If a community-wide change does occur, it will be difficult to ascertain which of the strategies might have contributed to this change. In all likelihood it is the variety of strategies occurring simultaneously in a community that has created change. Unless an experimental research design is adopted to help ascertain different levels of program intervention, it will not be possible to determine the crucial program components resulting in change.

**Step 3:
Identify
Resources
and
Constraints**

Throughout the evaluation, keep in mind available resources and constraints that may be encountered. Do you have the funds, time, and staff necessary to carry out the evaluation you have planned? Based on your answers, you need to consider what is realistic for each program. For example, if your program has volunteers or summer students, can some of their time be devoted to assisting you with the evaluation? If resources are limited, you may want to examine what is realistic to work on this year, as compared to starting with a multi-pronged evaluation. Based on the needs assessment results, the evaluation subcommittee may suggest several excellent evaluation strategies. However, available resources may require that you institute these interventions and their evaluation in phases.

You also need to identify factors that may work against conducting the evaluation. Participant characteristics, such as literacy and willingness to take a test or survey, will affect the evaluation. If you are collecting data from program records (for example, school dropout rates), you need to find out if that information is actually collected, accurate, and available. Does your staff support the evaluation efforts? Do you have the resources to analyze the data?

Consider other constraints within the community and the agency which may affect the research design, methods of data collection, and the specific questions that can be studied. Further, any legal restraints or agency regulations must be considered in

Example

Individual Program Objectives

Process Objectives	Outcome Objectives	Impact Objectives
• Deliver a five-part family life education program stressing abstinence and use of contraceptives (if sexually active) to 1,000 middle and high school students by June 30, 1994.	• Adolescents participating in the family life education program will increase their knowledge of effective contraceptives and decision-making skills by 25%.	• By January 1996, there will be a decrease in the time between on-set of sexual activity and adoption of a contraceptive method.
• Produce and distribute flyers and other promotional material by January 1, 1992 in order to inform teens of the programs and services at the teen community center.	• Adolescents enrolling in the counseling program at the teen community center will show a significant increase in self-esteem and decrease in depression scores at a six-month follow-up.	• By January 1997, the high school drop-out rate will have de-creased since the baseline needs assessment.
• Collaborate with the local job training program to establish a vocational planning program at the teen center by June 1, 1992	• Teens completing the vocational planning pro-gram at the teen community center will be able to state a vocational goal and the education and training they will need to obtain a job.	• By January, 1997, a minimum of 75% of participants in the job training program will be successfully placed in a job.
• By June 30, 1992 find potential funding sources and submit proposals for the co-location of a family planning specialist at the teen center.	• There will be a significant increase in the number of cross-referrals between the teen center and the family planning clinic as a result of the co-location of personnel.	• Contraceptive compli-ance and a significant reduction in unin-tended births will occur as a result of close follow-up of clinic clients by the family planning specialist as compared to a group of teen clients receiving traditional services.
	• Teen clients of the family planning clinic will show a significant increase in contraceptive compliance.	

Community-wide Effort Objectives

Process Objectives	Outcome Objectives	Impact Objectives
• By January 1, 1992 establish the Adoles-cent Health Services Network which will meet monthly in order to develop strategies to increase the coordi-nation of health and social services to adolescents.	• As compared to the baseline needs assessment survey, members of the community, (teens, parents, teachers, business leaders, and community non-profit agencies) will have a greater awareness of the incidence of teen pregnancy and the existing programs that address the problem.	• By January, 1996, decrease duplication and overlapping of health and social services to adoles-cents.
• By October 1992 generate a quarterly data report summariz-ing activities of all programs, including the total number of teens served by sex, age, ethnicity, and zip code of residence.	• Adolescents from key target areas will receive a compre-hensive array of services based on their individual-ized assessment plan.	• By January 1997, the rate of births to teens will have decreased since the baseline needs assessment.
	• Fewer adolescents from key target areas will remain without access to care.	• By January 1997, the high school drop-out rate will have de-creased significantly since the baseline needs assessment.

planning the evaluation. For example, many states require written parental consent before students are asked questions regarding sensitive or illegal behaviors. In such a situation, the evaluator may face a difficult choice: either obtaining responses to sensitive questions from a small and most likely biased sample (those who return consent forms); asking less intrusive questions; or seeking other pools of potential participants to whom the same restrictions do not apply – for example, out-of-school youth. See Worksheet 8-1 below to help identify resources and constraints.

Worksheet 8-1

Identifying Resources and Constraints

Directions: Identify the constraints you face and the resources available for implementing an evaluation. Complete this worksheet for each program you plan to evaluate as well as for the entire community-wide effort.

Target Population

Constraints	Resources
▪ *Many out-of-school youth are difficult to reach and trace*	▪ *Community is interested in reducing teen pregnancy rates*
	▪ *Strong interest in evaluation*

Environmental

Constraints	Resources
▪ *Some agencies concerned about the potential outcomes of the evaluation*	▪ *Consensus about the value of evaluation is well developed; staff involved in evaluation decisions*

Project Staff and Program

Constraints	Resources
▪ *Staff not trained in data collection*	▪ *Data items and evaluation questions are of interest to staff; staff are involved in developing data collection instruments; computerized data base is available for documenting data.*

Other

Constraints	Resources

Step 4: Specify What Information Is To Be Collected

It is necessary to specify how you are going to measure achievement of the objectives. From the program's measurable objectives, develop a list of evaluation questions. For example, an evaluation question for a life options program might be: "Did the program improve participants' awareness of how pregnancy would affect their ability to reach short- and long-term goals?" Since awareness is not something you can see, how can it be measured? You need to identify attitudes, behavioral intentions, or behaviors that would be indicators of awareness of the effects of pregnancy. You may decide that a good indicator would be the teenager's ability to identify steps necessary to reach a goal and to state how becoming pregnant would affect achievement of this goal. Thus, you would look for ways that this information could be collected from participants.

Information to be Collected for the Community-wide Evaluation

While you will gear your data collection to the individual objectives and activities of each separate component of your community-wide effort, you should also establish a core set of information items to be gathered across several programs. For example, you may have a family life education program for teenagers, both in schools and in alternative community settings. It would be helpful to identify the common items of the curriculum for each project when designing your evaluation tool, and collect similar data from each site.

The Sample Participant Summary Form (Worksheet 8-2) on page 228 represents information collected on each participant, by programs in the community-wide intervention. Using this form, every program can send demographic and participation information to a central data location. The agency or department managing the central database enters data into a computer and matches data for individuals participating in more than one program, to show how much of the intervention or "dosage" was received. These summary statistics are generated to show the total number of teens served; the number of participants per program; age, race, and school status distributions of participants, and so on.

As another example of data gathering, you might decide to do a random phone survey of youths to determine the impact of your entire community-based program on self-reported knowledge and attitudes toward adolescent pregnancy and pregnancy prevention, as well as on behavioral change. You will want to document the demographic profile of the respondents, including age, sex, and ethnicity, and assess whether these profiles are different for program participants and nonparticipants. For example, what is the background of male participants in the family life education parent/teen communication workshops, and what is the profile of non-participants? You will want to ask the respondents how many of the community interventions they participated in, and whether their level of participation affected their knowledge and attitude about adolescent pregnancy. Did they see the bus ads, attend a workshop, enroll at the teen center, and/or seek assistance at the family planning clinic? If so, do they feel any differently about delaying early childbearing? If you note that the respondents who participated in (or were exposed to) three or more community strategies

Worksheet 8-2   **Anytown Community Wide Teen Pregnancy Prevention Program**
Sample Participant Summary Form

Identification Number: __ __ __ __

Age: __ __   Birth Date: __ __ / __ __ / __ __

Education: __ __

0	no schooling	8	completed eighth grade
1	completed first grade	9	completed ninth grade
2	completed second grade	10	completed tenth grade
3	completed third grade	11	completed eleventh grade
4	completed fourth grade	12	graduated high school
5	completed fifth grade	13	completed GED/CHSPE
6	completed sixth grade	14	schooling above high school
7	completed seventh grade	99	unknown

School Status: __

1 currently attending school
2 not currently attending school

Race/Ethnicity: __ __

1	White	5	Chinese	8	Southeast Asian
2	Black	6	Japanese	9	Undeclared
3	Hispanic	7	Filipino	10	Other: ___
4	American Indian				

Family Life Education: __

1 attended middle school FLE program
2 attended high school FLE program
3 attended FLE program at Teen Community Center
4 attended FLE program elsewhere (specify:_____)
5 has not attended a FLE program

Teen Community Center:

A. Job Training Program: __

1 completed job training program
2 began job training program but did not complete
3 did not participate in job training program

B. Personal Counseling: __

1 received personal counseling (number of sessions: __ __)
2 did not receive personal counseling

C. Peer Tutoring for School: __

1 received peer tutoring services
2 did not receive peer tutoring services

D. Recreation Program: __

1	participated in a recreational program	6	crafts classes
2	evening open center hours	7	camping outing
3	afternoon open center hours	8	pool tournament
4	basketball tournament	9	did not participate in
5	life skills class		a recreation program

E. Received personal family planning counseling: __

1 received personal family planning counseling
2 did not receive personal family planning counseling

F. Referred to teen clinic for clinical family planning services: __

1 was referred to teen family planning clinic
2 was not referred to teen family planning clinic

School-based Health Clinic:

A. Received personal family planning counseling: __

1 received personal family planning counseling
2 did not receive personal family planning counseling

B. Referred to teen clinic for clinical family planning services: __

1 received personal family planning counseling
2 did not receive personal family planning counseling

C. Received personal counseling: __

1 received personal counseling (number of sessions: __ __)
2 did not receive personal counseling

D. Used clinic's medical services: __

1 used clinic's medical services (e.g. athletic physical, illness)
2 did not use clinic's medical services

Teen Family Planning Clinic: __

1 received family planning services
2 did not receive family planning services

If received services, referred by: __

1 School-based Health Clinic counselor
2 Teen Community Center counselor
3 FLE teacher
4 media (flyers, posters, radio, etc.)
5 friend
6 other:_____

have a more positive attitude toward the delay of pregnancy or are consistently using contraceptives (if they are sexually active) then you may be able to argue for continuing a variety of strategies. It is important to realize, however, that even if respondents may have been exposed to the program, they may not have been aware that it was part of a community-wide effort.

If one objective of the community-wide program is to improve coordination among youth-serving agencies, documentation could include data on whether an adolescent health and social services network has been established, how it is functioning, whether letters of agreement between participating agencies have been established, and whether a centralized data system to track clients through the system has been implemented.

On the following page is an example of a work sheet showing the type of information that is needed to answer specific questions:

Example   ## Indicators of Project Goals and Objectives

Objective: The multi-agency sponsored Teen Center will provide the community's adolescents with after-school job preparation and training programs.

Evaluation Question 1: Did the Teen Center provide after school programs?

Process Indicator: Identify which programs were actually implemented, and document how many agencies participated in program development and the extent of their participation.

Evaluation Question 2: Did teens participate in these programs?

Process Indicator: Count how many teens participated in each program (job skills training, family life education, etc.).

Evaluation Question 3: What was the result of participating in these programs?

Outcome Indicator: Document the percentage of teens in the job training program who had jobs six months after completing it.

Impact Indicator: Follow up these trainees to see how many continued to be employed 12 and 18 months after concluding the program.

Objective: As a result of the extensive community-wide effort, the rate of births to teens will decrease significantly as compared to the rate documented in the baseline needs assessment.

Evaluation Question 4: Did expansion of family planning sites accompanied by an increased level of outreach and follow-up for teenagers contribute to a reduced risk of adolescent pregnancy in the community?

Process Indicator: Document whether there was a significant increase in the number of adolescents who receive family planning services.

Outcome Indicator: Document whether there was an increase in the level of self-reported contraceptive compliance among adolescents attending clinics.

Evaluation Question 5: Did the teen birth rate decrease?

Impact Indicator: Yearly county birth rates by age of mother.

Note: As you review your own project goals and objectives, assess what process, outcome and impact indicators are most appropriate for your community.

**Step 5:
Choose the
Evaluation
Design**

The program evaluation design determines when data are collected and from whom information is gathered. An evaluation design is needed for each component of the overall community-wide plan. For example, while a pre- and post-intervention assessment may work well for an educational program, different methods may be necessary to assess the effect of a media campaign. Whether you are designing an evaluation to assess the impact of a community-wide program, or the evaluation of a specific program, there are different designs that you can use:

• Post-assessment only

• One-group pre- and post-assessment

• Pre- and post-test comparison group

• Time series design

It is also important to establish a comparison group so that you can determine if the program intervention really made a difference. Five ways to establish a comparison group include:

• Simple random assignment

• Systematic sampling

• Participant or peer-generated groups

• Matching by unit

• Use of existing data sets

The following designs will help assess the outcomes and impact of the programs. Consider the intent of the evaluation as well as the constraints and resources in deciding what design best fits your situation. Following the explanation of each of the four designs is a diagram with the following symbols: X represents the treatment given to the experimental group, the effects of which are to be assessed; O refers to an observation or measure that may take the form of a questionnaire, interview, etc. Each row of symbols represents a different group of people. The order of symbols from left to right indicates earlier to later events. Symbols in the same column indicate different groups participating in the event at the same time.

	Observation 1		Observation 2
Treatment Group *(receiving the intervention)*	O	X	O
Control Group *(receiving traditional approach/no intervention)*	O		O
	Pre-test observation	**Program intervention**	**Post-test observation**

Post-assessment			Observation 1
Only	**Treatment Group**	X	O

In this design, program participants receive an assessment (survey, questionnaire, interview, etc.) after they have participated in a program. The design can measure the level of knowledge, skills or reported behavior of participants after a program has been conducted. However, there is no way to determine if this group has improved as a result of the program or would have improved to the same degree even if no program had been provided.

One-group Pre- and		Observation 1		Observation 2
Post-assessment	**Treatment Group**	O	X	O

In this design, information is collected prior to participation in the program, and again after participating in the program. By measuring the difference between pre- and post-assessment measures, you can determine the amount of change that took place. However, because there is no comparison group, this design does not account for the possibility that the measured change might have occurred without the program.

Pre-test/Post-test		Observation 1		Observation 2
Comparison Group	**Treatment Group**	O	X	O
	Comparison Group	O		O

This design is the same as the one-group pre-test/post-test except that participants are assigned to the treatment or comparison group. This design is strengthened because the comparison group allows you to rule out the possibility that the measured change might have occurred without the program. However, finding a comparison group or assigning individuals to a control group can be difficult.

Time Series Design	**Treatment Group**	O	O	O	X	O	O	O

In this design, observations are taken before, during and after a program is introduced. In this way, you can determine if the program had any effect on the trend of whatever you are measuring. This is a good design to use when you have enough time and resources to collect the data or, even better, if the data that you are interested in are already being collected, for example, as part of ongoing clinic records. Time periods between observations must be equal.

For example, you may want to track rates of births to teens, or high school dropout rates, both before the community-wide effort began and several times after the program has been implemented. One would want to collect data after the program has been operating for a sufficient period of time in order to assess whether there have been any changes and whether the program has had any measurable impact. It would also be important to monitor the full array of program interventions throughout the time that data are collected to assure their continuous availability.

Establishing a Control or Comparison Group

Control or comparison groups greatly strengthen evaluation designs because they allow you to compare the treatment group to one that did not receive the intervention(s). (A control group is established by random assignment, while a comparison group is established by nonrandom assignment.) A control or comparison group is used to help determine whether program participants actually improved as a result of the program, rather than for some other reason. This is particularly helpful when you are working with young people who may change frequently merely through the process of maturing. Without observing a comparison or control group you cannot account for the possibility that measured change in knowledge, attitudes, or behavior might have occurred in the absence of the program. However, selecting such a group is often a difficult choice in community settings where it would require that services are denied to one group. Rather than assigning a group to receive no services, you may wish to provide them with an alternative treatment. This can work well if you are trying to improve upon an existing service or program. For example, you may compare a new style of counseling teens to the standard counseling protocol. This design is further strengthened by randomly assigning individuals to the new and alternative intervention.

Comparison groups may be more difficult to select when conducting a community-wide evaluation. A community can act as its own comparison community if adequate documentation exists on the anticipated outcome measurements (such as school dropout rates) before the intervention(s) have been implemented. Documented change then can be monitored with the introduction of the different interventions. However, one should be cautious in interpreting these data and drawing conclusions about the causality of interventions and outcomes, as some other factors may also be contributing to changes in the community. For example, with the onset of AIDS, new health education campaigns have emerged emphasizing the need for condoms. These powerful messages could have a secondary affect on the community's incidence of sexually transmitted diseases and the incidence of adolescent births.

If the community is large, and there are several areas which are comparable, both in terms of the numbers of adolescents at risk of pregnancy and the incidence of adolescent births and school dropouts, the community may find that it only has sufficient funding to implement and test new interventions in a specifically targeted neighborhood. In such a situation, the chosen indicators (outcomes) may be compared for the target community and for neighborhoods that did not receive a new infusion of effort.

A third kind of comparison involves the use of comparable communities that have parallel levels of adolescent pregnancy related problems. It is important that the communities be as similar as possible and that there is monitoring of both communities to assess whether any unanticipated changes may impact the outcomes. For example, a new job training program in the control community may impact the adolescent employment status and in turn affect teen birth rates.

In any of these situations, it is important to assess whether the adopted interventions are of sufficient strength to impact the planned outcomes. Even when a family life education, health, or social service program is excellent, staff must recognize other factors, such as high levels of unemployment and poverty, that may hamper community change.

The key issue in establishing a comparison group is whether or not it adequately controls for the effects of other factors that might produce or explain the observed impact. In order to assert that your program did make a change, your comparison group should be as similar as possible to your program participants in characteristics that might affect the changes you are trying to produce. Although many times demographic profiles such as age, sex, and ethnicity are relied on to match intervention and comparison groups, it is important to obtain other measures. For example, what is the incidence of school truancy and school dropout at each site? How many participants live with only one parent? What other community services are being provided on-site in each of the schools? It is also important to note that there are few communities today which have a total absence of programs, so even the comparison group will have some level of service provision.

Random Assignment

Random assignment of participants to the control and experimental groups, in evaluations in which the experimental group receives an intervention and the other does not, is the most desirable method for establishing comparison groups. In random sampling, each person has an equal chance of being selected for either group, and assignment to either group is independent of any other event in the selection process. It is the best method to ensure internal validity, meaning that the conclusions derived from the evaluation accurately reflect what has gone on in the study. Random assignment may help to counteract some of the factors that may threaten the validity of the evaluation, such as the following:

• Unexpected events may occur during the course of the evaluation, such as a statewide media effort on teen pregnancy.

• Young people will grow and mature, regardless of the program.

• There may be a bias in how people are selected and assigned to the study group.

• Participants may decide to drop out of the evaluation in numbers that can skew the results.

- The process of testing and retesting may influence responses.

- There is a statistical likelihood of "regression to the mean," which means that people who start out in some extreme position will tend to move toward the average.

Random assignment will at least increase the likelihood that these factors will be distributed fairly evenly between the two groups. For example, participants in both groups should mature at about the same rate, so you will know that differences between groups are not likely to be the result of maturation alone.

The following kinds of sampling approaches are most applicable to a single program evaluation, but are not as feasible for a community-wide intervention:

- **Simple random sampling** assignment can be easily performed using a computer-generated randomization list. To use the randomization table in Appendix 8-1, just write participants' names on the roster and read off from the column the number of the group to which the individual is assigned. The "Roster for Random Assignment" can be used to randomize to 2, 3, 4 or 5 groups.

- In **systematic sampling**, people are chosen at regular intervals. For example you could assign every other person attending a clinic to the counseling services and the rest to the standard services. Selecting from a list or pool of individuals who enter a program in no particular pattern will most likely result in a random sample.

- **Participant or peer-generated groups** are established by having participants identify one or two friends or neighbors much like themselves in age, sex, race, socioeconomic status, etc. Participants are asked to provide the names and phone numbers of these people, who in turn will be contacted by program staff. This can be a very convenient way to obtain a comparison group. Drawbacks of this method are that participants may not wish to identify comparison friends; and they may discuss program content with the friends before project staff contact them, possibly creating a "spillover" effect of the program content. Thus, this comparison group has limitations.

- **Matching by unit.** You may have the opportunity to match data in a neighborhood or school where a program is being provided, with data from a comparable neighborhood or school where the intervention(s) you are testing have not been introduced. Identify approximately the same number of individuals as there are in the treatment group, and match them by age, sex, race, and any other characteristic that might affect results, such as exposure to previous family life education curricula provided in the schools. It is important to note what is being offered to the nonparticipants, as you may find that the two groups' outcomes may not be significantly different, but the new program is more cost-efficient.

- **Existing data sets.** Consider using existing data sets for your evaluation when it is not possible to use a comparison group, or when funds for data collection are limited. Researchers who have developed large national data bases have provided their data to a centralized Data Archive on Adolescent Pregnancy and Pregnancy Prevention in Los Altos, California (see Sociometrics, General Resource Directory, page 268). You may be able to compare evaluation results to those catalogued in the archive by comparing the composition of your groups (by demographic indicators) and the incidence of adolescent births, school dropout levels, etc., to a national sample (Card and Reagan, 1989). Some potential drawbacks are the differences in the years data was collected for the different studies; geographical differences; and the difficulty of identifying a data set that will allow for matching minorities, particularly specific Southeast Asian and Central American groups.

Step 6: Choose the Data Collection Method

Select the most appropriate method for collecting information, and construct the necessary instruments. Again, data collection approaches may vary depending on whether you are planning to conduct an evaluation of your community-wide effort, or you are specifically focusing on one type of program intervention.

Five data collection options are:

- Questionnaires

- Interviews

- Direct observation

- Existing program records

- Public records

If possible, you should use multiple methods of data collection, since one method may detect what another cannot. Furthermore, if you find results to be consistent for each method used, you have an additional indication that your evaluation results are reliable. Worksheet 8-3, Identifying Methods of Data Collection, is provided to assist you in determining the optimum approach for collecting information on each type of program.

Questionnaires and Surveys

Questionnaires are the most common method of data collection used in health education interventions, whether they are used in a specific program or in a community-wide intervention. Questionnaires can be answered anonymously, can be administered to many people simultaneously, and can impose uniformity on the information obtained by requesting the same information from all respondents. On the other hand, written questionnaires do not provide much depth of information, they are impersonal,

Worksheet 8-3   # Identifying Methods of Data Collection

Directions: For each of your indicators (information collected to answer evaluation questions), check off the method(s) of data collection you will use. Consider both the internal and external constraints your program faces and the available resources to resolve these potential barriers to evaluation.

Example:

Objective: Improve the knowledge of adolescents age 14-17 regarding teen pregnancy.

Question: Do program participants know the consequences of unintended teen pregnancy?

Indicator: Teens will identify three consequences of an unintended pregnancy

Methods of Data Collection:

☐ Written post-test　☑ Written pre- and post-test
☑ Verbal test　☐ Mail or telephone follow-up
☐ Records　☑ Graded homework assignment
☐ Observation　☐ Other:_____

Objective: _____

Question: _____

Indicator: _____

Methods of Data Collection:

☐ Written post-test　☐ Written pre- and post-test
☐ Verbal test　☐ Mail or telephone follow-up
☐ Records　☐ Graded homework assignment
☐ Observation　☐ Other:_____

Objective: _____

Question: _____

Indicator: _____

Methods of Data Collection:

☐ Written post-test　☐ Written pre- and post-test
☐ Verbal test　☐ Mail or telephone follow-up
☐ Records　☐ Graded homework assignment
☐ Observation　☐ Other:_____

Objective:_____

Question:_____

Indicator:_____

Methods of Data Collection:

☐ Written post-test　☐ Written pre- and post-test
☐ Verbal test　☐ Mail or telephone follow-up
☐ Records　☐ Graded homework assignment
☐ Observation　☐ Other:_____

and they may be read carelessly or be misunderstood. They are also difficult to administer to people who are illiterate or anxious about taking tests. Standard question formats are: fill-in-the-blank, multiple choice, true/false, rank order, and Likert-type items. All questionnaires should incorporate adequate written instructions.

- **Fill-in-the-blank** is the primary open-ended format used in questionnaires. An open-ended question is one in which respondents are asked to provide their own answer to the question. While this type of question provides flexibility and may get close to a respondent's feelings, it is also more difficult to score and analyze.

- **Multiple choice** items are closed-ended. That is, the respondent is asked to select an answer among a list provided on the questionnaire. This format is relatively easy to answer and to score.

- **True/False** items request the respondent to indicate whether a statement is true (correct) or false (incorrect). We also recommend adding the category of "not sure" to prevent respondents giving half-true answers. This format can only be used when measuring knowledge of facts that are clearly right or wrong. It can also be used to give program participants statements about which they can either agree or disagree.

- **Rank order** items require the respondent to arrange a series of responses to a question in order of perceived importance. The respondent may be asked to list aspects of a topic in order of priority from least to most important, or from most to least in importance. For example, the questionnaire may ask the adolescent to rank in priority order the activities sponsored by the local teen center.

- **Likert scale**-type items present the respondent with a statement and ask whether the individual "strongly agrees," "agrees," "disagrees," "strongly disagrees," or is "undecided." This question format allows one to determine how strongly a person favors or disfavors a certain attitude or value. It can also be used to ascertain how often a person engages in certain behavior. In this case, the range of possible answers may include "always," "often," "sometimes," "hardly ever," and "never."

Using Existing Questionnaires

It is not necessary to reinvent the wheel when you construct an evaluation questionnaire. If you find appropriate questions on another test used in the field, incorporate them in your questionnaire. Call the program or agency that developed the questionnaire and discuss their experiences in using it. Most agencies will be cooperative in allowing others to use their tests. Only in rare cases will you find restrictions in the use of a questionnaire. Just be sure all of the items you incorporate reflect your program's evaluation objectives. Always pilot-test a tool even if it has been used successfully elsewhere, or previously in your program, but with a different objective. This is particularly important if the program(s) are attempting to reach a different target population. It should be noted that the closest indicator measurements available to evaluators may be behavioral intent questions in which respondents are asked a series of questions regarding behaviors they anticipate they may engage in and under what circumstances they might engage in them.

Principles for Writing Good Questionnaires

The following principles are applicable to questionnaires that are used in testing a specific program within the community-wide plan, or in assessing the impact of the total community-wide intervention.

- Be sure the instrument actually measures your objectives, rather than whether the clients approved of the program.

  Devote the majority of the items to demonstrating attitude, knowledge, and behavior changes instead of participants' reaction to the program. Too often there is an implied reasoning that if people enjoyed the program it will impact their behavior. Rely on client satisfaction questions only if you are trying to improve the program's services. You should also be aware that changing knowledge and attitudes will not necessarily be translated into behavioral changes. Thus, if your program objectives are geared to behavioral change, do not devote the majority of your questionnaire to knowledge and attitude items.

- Ask questions only on material that has been presented.

  Do not ask a question on a topic that was not covered in a program. If you find that the information reflected in any of the questionnaire items was not specifically covered during the program, delete that question from pre- and post-test analysis.

- Order questions from least to most threatening.

  Asking a very personal or sensitive question first (e.g., "Are you currently sexually active?") may cause a respondent to feel uncomfortable with the questionnaire, and not answer questions truthfully.

- Always provide a clear set of instructions.

  If possible, both verbal and written instructions for completing the questionnaire should be given. As a way to reduce test-taking anxiety, you may want to state that the purpose of the questionnaire is to test the program, not the participants.

- Make sure items are clear and precise.

  Let the person completing the questionnaire know exactly what is being asked. Asking respondents to complete very general sentences, such as "I think

_____" may not provide you with useful evaluation information. Also avoid questions that ask the respondents what they knew or thought before the program or presentation; it is difficult for individuals to assess their level of knowledge or comfort retroactively. For example, ask parents how comfortable they feel talking with their children about sex before the program, during the baseline survey. Don't ask them at a post-intervention assessment to recall how they felt before the program.

- Make response categories exhaustive and mutually exclusive.

Responses presented as choices in the questionnaire should include all possible alternatives. For example, if participants are asked: "What method of birth control do you use?" and the questionnaire only provides the answers: "a. birth control pill; b. diaphragm; c. condom; d. sponge," a person who uses natural family planning, withdrawal, or multiple methods or who does not use any birth control could not respond. It is often useful to include a category labelled "Other (please specify _____)" for nonfactual questions or "I'm not sure" for knowledge-type questions.

- Avoid double-barreled questions.

Do not ask for a single response to more than one question, for example: "Did you learn a lot from this program and would you recommend it to your friends?" In this case, participants may have learned a lot, but still feel hesitant to suggest that others attend.

- Avoid negative items.

Negative items (using words like "not" or "don't") may open the question to misinterpretation. For example, if asked to disagree or agree with the statement, "Parents should not talk with their children about sex," an individual may skip over the word "not" or misunderstand how to respond.

- Use appropriate vocabulary.

Use only terms that you are absolutely sure will be understood by your respondents. If potentially unfamiliar words are used you may want to put a more common or lay term in parenthesis. For example, to clarify the word "condom," you may follow it with words such as rubber, protection, or sheath. You may need to conduct informal interviews with members of the target group (both adults and teens) in order to learn what vocabulary is best understood by each of the populations you are trying to reach.

- Make questions interesting.

Using pictures and scenarios can make the questionnaire informative and attractive. For example, you could present the following scenario:

"Your teenager has started going steady with a classmate. As far as you know, your child has never been intimate before with a boy/girlfriend. You don't think they are at the point of having sexual relations. You feel very strongly that your child should not have sex until he/she is older."

After presenting the scenario, you can ask parents questions such as "What would you do if you were the parent in this situation?" or "Name two ways you could raise the topic of sexuality in a conversation with your teenager if you found yourself in this situation."

Adding pictures can make questions more fun, and easier to answer. The faces below can be used with attitude questions such as: "Sex education in schools helps prevent teenage pregnancy."

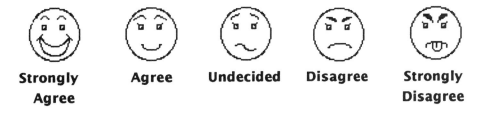

| Strongly Agree | Agree | Undecided | Disagree | Strongly Disagree |

- Make items match the intervention.

There should be proportional correspondence between the length of time devoted to a specific topic in the program or curriculum and the number of total questions on that topic included in the final evaluation instrument.

- Be prepared to pilot and revise!

Even the best questionnaire may need to be revised after you have conducted a pilot test of it. Revisions may also be necessary as the program matures and the target audience or the programs change. A community-wide plan, and the programs geared to its implementation, are bound to change and adapt over time. Be sure that the tools continue to measure the objectives of the intervention(s) you're evaluating.

Interviews

There are certain advantages to having questionnaires administered by interviewers, either at the project site, the participant's home, another convenient location, or by telephone. Interviews have the advantage of flexibility. The interviewer can probe for answers, thus decreasing the number of "don't knows" or "no answers." Interviews can also be used to obtain information from people who have a low level of literacy or those who are anxious about taking a test. However, verbal interviews are time-consuming, and the interviewer may influence the respondent's answers by the manner in which questions are asked, through body language, tone of voice, and subtle changes in wording of questions. Staff require special training in interviewing to assure unbiased, accurate results. If you hire outside interviewers, it is especially important to monitor their work (for example, by contacting a sampling of people who have been interviewed, to verify that the interview took place). The following suggestions are designed to assist you in developing effective interview procedures.

* Make special arrangements for adolescents.

   If you plan to conduct interviews with adolescents, you will often need to gain entry via a parent. Establish a confidential place in which to hold the interview. If the teenager will be talking by telephone from home, it is important to assure that privacy is possible. If not, consider another setting.

* The interviewer should be familiar enough with the instrument to be able to read it without stumbling over words and phrases.

   Make sure the interviewer has adequate time to review the survey instrument and practice using the questionnaire before the initial interviews take place.

* Interviewers should be prepared to probe for responses when answers given are inappropriate or incomplete.

   Probes are also necessary in eliciting responses to open-ended questions. For example, when asked about the usefulness of a family communication workshop, an interviewee might simply reply: "It was pretty helpful." Possible probes might be: "In what ways?", "How was it helpful?", or "Anything else?" Sometimes the best probe is silence. The respondent may fill in the pause with additional comments.

* For some personal questions, including those pertaining to income, develop a separate card that shows the respondents ranges of responses, so that they can just select a letter representing the answer, instead of answering with specific information.

   For example: Please review the following answers to the question, "What is your monthly income?" (show card) A. less than $500/month; B. $500-$1000/month; C. $1001-$1500/month; D. more than $1500/month.

* It is important to record a response to an open-ended question as accurately as possible.

Attempts should not be made to summarize or paraphrase an answer. If this is done, much of the rich detail is lost, and the meaning may be changed. With the permission of the interviewee, the session can be taped and later transcribed. This allows the interviewer more freedom to observe, and makes the respondent more comfortable. While taping may not be feasible for every interview, taping even a sample of interviews will help in capturing the interactions. Taping is also useful in monitoring the quality of the data being collected as it allows you to assess the consistency of the interviewer's notes by comparing them with the conversation that has taken place.

• Train interviewers to be as uniform as possible in data collection methods.

Group training is preferable to individual training. The training session should include the following activities:

1. Describe what the study is all about.

2. Discuss general guidelines and procedures.

3. Review the instrument – question by question.

4. Have trainees practice administering the interview to each other.

• Document the numbers of individuals who decline to participate in the interview and their reasons for declining.

Ideally, a profile of characteristics of non-participants should be compared to that of participants to assess differences between groups. Make extra efforts to include individuals who may not be traditionally included, such as school drop-outs.

• Beware of the sampling problems inherent in telephone surveys.

While telephone interviews are a convenient approach to gathering data, be aware of potential limitations. First, while telephones are commonplace, the sample is limited to those who have phones in their home. Individuals targeted for community interventions may not all have the economic means to pay for a telephone. Second, if you are sampling from a local phone directory, all the people who have requested that their numbers not be published will be excluded from the sample. Telephone surveys, however, can be a reliable way of collecting data.

Existing Program Records

Sources of data that reflect the effectiveness of the program may already exist in the form of program records. You may be able to extract information for the evaluation from records that are kept for purposes other than program evaluation. These can be valuable if they are systematically maintained over an extensive period of time. Measurement sources may include sign-in sheets, records of calls for information, or records of consultation. From these records you can obtain:

- Data on numbers of clients served

- Number of visits made

- Amount of contact between the program and participant

- Needs of the population

- Characteristics of the population the program is serving

While program records may allow you to gather data conveniently and inexpensively, they have inherent limitations. The records may not supply all the information you are seeking, although you may find that they provide you with valuable insights as to how the program is functioning. You also must assess how completely and accurately records are being maintained. As the community-wide interventions are implemented, program record keeping may be revised to gather additional information. For example, the numbers and kinds of interagency referrals may be added to the program data bank and help document an important outcome objective for the community.

The chart review on page 245 (Worksheet 8-4) is an example of a data collection form used for abstracting data from the charts of a community clinic. It was used as one component of an evaluation of new counseling and case management services for the clinic's teen clients. The information helped document whether additional drug and alcohol counseling should be part of the services available onsite or through referral.

Public Records

Public records such as census data, governmental reports, and data maintained by health and school departments will probably be the primary source of data used to evaluate the impact of the community-wide plan. Monitoring adolescent birth trends for the targeted census areas is a useful approach to assessing the overall impact of the program. The interventions need to be of sufficient strength and duration to anticipate that the overall trends will change. In addition, a variety of external factors, such as changes in the demographic composition of a community, may also affect the results. For example, an influx of Southeast Asian refugees, who have cultural traditions of early marriage and childbearing, may affect birth trends as well as the overall age composition of the community. Check to see whether the numbers of adolescents ages 17 and under are remaining the same, or if there has been an age shift in the community. In order to assess existing trends, compare birth data for several years before and after initiation of different interventions. Note that in the case study from South Carolina (page 246), changes in pregnancy rates did not show up until two years after the first year of implementation.

Worksheet 8-4

Case Management Project:
Chart Review

Patient No.: __ __ __ __ __ __   Reviewer's Initials: _____

Date of Initial Visit: __ __/__ __/__ __   Age (at initial visit): __ __   Sex: [1] F [2]
                         month day   year

Ethnic Group: [1] White   [6] Filipino

                  [2] Black   [7] Other Asian_____

                  [3] Am Indian   [8] Hispanic

                  [4] Chinese   [9] Missing

                  [5] Japanese   [10] Other_____

Age at first intercourse: __ __

Smokes cigarettes: [1] Yes   [2] No   [9] Missing

Drinks alcohol: [1] Yes   [2] No   [9] Missing

Uses drugs: [1] Yes   [2] No   [9] Missing

If Yes what drugs:_____

Has previously had an STD: [1] Yes   [2] No   [9] Missing

Number of pregnancies (or partner's pregnancies) before initiating care at clinic:____

Did client return for annual exam 12-13 months after first clinic visit? [1] Yes [2] No

Number of pregnancies (or of partner) since initial clinic visit:____

Birth data can also be studied in conjunction with data from other sources. For example, as part of the Center for Population Option's national evaluation of school-based health clinics, Dr. Doug Kirby provided a local health department with a listing of all high school students who attended a school where a school-based clinic operated. Using a computerized data bank, the health department compared that list with a list of adolescents who had given birth. After comparing the lists, the health department reported the number (but not the names) of individuals who had been enrolled in the school and who had given birth during the past five years. Thus, the impact of the program on those in contact with the intervention could be studied. Due to confidentiality requirements, it was not possible in this case to provide a list differentiating those students who used the school-based clinic from those who did not. Thus, this analysis compared the overall impact of the clinic on the total student body.

Observations   Conducting observations of participants attending the health, education, and social services programs is another useful evaluation method that can be used in conjunction with the methods previously reviewed. Observations can help document a person's ability to apply information in life-like situations, can provide information when other methods are not possible, and can provide both qualitative and quantitative data. However, observations are a more difficult way to collect valid and reliable data, and they are subject to personal interpretation and bias of the observer. Long periods of training and experience may be required for the observer. It is helpful to have a person who is not normally involved with the facility conduct the observations from the side or back of the room. In highly structured observations, an observer records a

Example

South Carolina's Adolescent Pregnancy Prevention Program: A Case Study*

A school and community-based education program was implemented in South Carolina from 1982 to 1987. Intervention messages were targeted simultaneously at parents, teachers, church representatives, community leaders, and children enrolled in the public school system. The primary behavioral objectives of the program were to postpone initial voluntary sexual intercourse among never-married teens and preteens and to promote the consistent use of effective contraception among those who are sexually active. The impact objective was to reduce the occurrence of unintended pregnancy among never-married teens and preteens.

The western portion of a South Carolina county received the intervention, while the eastern portion which served as a comparison group did not. The entire county population is demographically homogeneous. Because of the potential spillover between residents of the county, three additional similar South Carolina counties were selected as comparison groups.

Trends in annual age-specific estimated pregnancy rates (EPR) for females age 14-17 years were used to assess the impact of the intervention. There was a sharp reduction in the number of pregnancies in the intervention area of the county after 1983, a lesser reduction in the nonintervention area, and little change in the comparison counties.

Annual Age-Specific Estimated Pregnancy Rates (EPRs) for Females Ages 14-17 Years**

	YEAR				
Geographic Area	**1981**	**1982**	**1983**	**1984**	**1985**
Intervention portion of target county	54.1	67.1	61.7	25.1	25.1
Comparison portion of target county	63.9	69.7	63.1	58.8	46.0
Comparison county 1	47.9	57.9	40.4	56.3	60.2
Comparison county 2	37.9	31.7	44.2	48.6	53.7
Comparison county 3	32.5	44.9	45.1	50.3	54.9

**EPR=(live births + fetal deaths + induced abortions)/1000 female population
* Based on research conducted by Vincent, Clearie, and Schluchter, (1987).

defined set of behaviors on a checklist, or according to a pre-written coding system. In less structured situations, the observer records a continuous description of the behaviors seen.

The following is a sample observation form which was used in evaluating a community birth control education program. Students were observed doing role plays at the conclusion of a five-part education series. Items one and two are individual measures of two students role playing a situation in which two teens are discussing birth control. Items three through six assess the group of participants in a discussion of myths concerning pregnancy.

Example

Observation Instrument
Family Life Education Program

Date:__ __/__ __/__ __   Location:_____

Name of Observer:_____

Observations of Role Play

Check the appropriate box for each member of the group taking part in the role-playing exercise. If more than one group participates, use another sheet.

Scenario: Couple discussing forms of birth control.

	Participant One	Participant Two
1. Participant states:		
a. no appropriate alternatives to the birth control pill	☐	☐
b. 1 appropriate alternative to the birth control pill	☐	☐
c. at least 2 appropriate alternatives to the birth control pill	☐	☐
d. at least 3 appropriate alternatives to the birth control pill	☐	☐
e. at least 4 appropriate alternatives to the birth control pill	☐	☐

2. Participant correctly identifies a minimum of two locations
where birth control can be obtained.   ☐ Yes   ☐ No

Discussion of Myths

Myth: You cannot get pregnant:	Most of group agrees	Mixed opinion	Most of group disagrees
3. the first time you have intercourse	☐	☐	☐
4. if you use certain positions	☐	☐	☐
5. if the male withdraws	☐	☐	☐

6. Group involvement:
   a. **Very good.** Group was very receptive; active discussion.   ☐
   b. **Fair.** Seemed interested, but did not participate much in discussion.   ☐
   c. **Poor.** Inattentive, resistant to dialogue, seemed bored.   ☐

7. Anecdotal information indicating group/individual involvement:_____

_____

_____

Step 7:
Test and
Refine
Procedures
and Tools

It is not easy to plan an evaluation and design data collection tools that will provide a community with the evaluation information needed. Always plan for time to pre-test forms, questionnaires, and data collection procedures. You may find that some questions are not clear or that you cannot obtain access to information that exists in public records. For example, while you may want to track the teen pregnancy rate in your community, you may find that the information you need on the rate of induced abortions and miscarriages is either not available or incomplete. You need all three components — births, abortions, and miscarriages — to calculate the pregnancy rate. As an alternative indicator measurement for an impact evaluation, you may have to track age-specific birthrates instead. In addition, you need to document whether the quality of data and the reporting of that data have changed (for example, whether school attendance record keeping has improved with the introduction of a computerized system). If data quality changes occur simultaneously with the introduction of the proposed interventions, the community will not be able to disentangle the effects of the program from the effects of changes in reporting the data.

Questionnaires should be pilot-tested on a sample of participants as similar as possible to the individuals who will be participating in the program. Be sure to elicit feedback from these individuals on the clarity of the questions and the appropriateness of the vocabulary. It can be useful to have them tell you what the questions mean in their own words. If you choose to conduct interviews, be certain that interviewers are adequately trained in collecting information in a consistent and complete manner.

During the pilot, you may also find you are unable to gain access to information in public documents, or the quality of data is poor. The pilot phase will allow you to refine data collection procedures and/or identify alternative approaches. Time is always necessary to iron out unexpected glitches in the evaluation plan.

Step 8:
Collect Data

The quality of data being collected must be closely monitored. If several people are collecting data make sure that they are collecting and coding information in the same way and are following procedures prescribed in the evaluation manual. This monitoring should occur throughout the data collection process. It is a crucial element in the overall evaluation because the value of the conclusions about the findings is based on the quality of the data.

Confidentiality of Data

Respondents need to be protected from the possible emotional discomfort of answering certain questions. If you are working within an organization or institution, such as a university, you will probably need to obtain permission to conduct your evaluation from an institutional review board, which exists to protect the rights of individuals participating in research or evaluation studies.

It is also the responsibility of the evaluating agency to prevent anyone from using the information inappropriately. Thus, it is important to keep all information confidential.

Completed questionnaires should be identified by code numbers instead of names. In order to give "informed consent", potential participants should be told: 1) the purpose of the data collection, 2) how the information will be used, 3) that data will be kept confidential and in many cases will be collected anonymously, 4) that data from all interviews or questionnaires will be summarized rather than reported on individuals, and 5) that they have the right to refuse to participate and may refuse to answer any particular question without endangering their right to receive any services.

You may wish to hand participants a list of these rights along with the name and phone number of a person they may contact at a later date if they have questions. If you want to obtain signed consent you can leave space at the bottom of the list for respondents to sign after they have read and understood their rights and have agreed to participate. One copy of this consent form should be left with the participant and one copy should be kept in the files. In some settings, it may not be feasible to distribute a written consent (for example, when conducting a clinic chart review) but careful documentation of the informed consent process is still important.

A common data collection design includes pre- and post-program assessments, which trace specific people through time. However, putting individual's names on questionnaires may put their confidentiality in jeopardy. An alternative is to assign an identification number to each individual in the program and use these as identifiers on the data collection tools. The numbers can be ones you assign or ones the participant makes up. They should be easy to remember since they will not change throughout the course of the program. For example, one easy-to-recall code is comprised of participant's date of birth and the first two digits of his/her street address.

**Step 9:
Analyze Data**

Data analysis procedures help to organize and summarize the data. There are two primary ways to analyze data: through descriptive statistics or through inferential statistics. Descriptive statistics are representative measurements, such as the average and the variability that occurs from the mean. These numbers allow one to make sense of the information that has been collected and to evaluate the effectiveness of the program in reaching its goals. For example, the mean score for a survey could be 15, but the group variability may show that half of the group gets within that average score by two points. That is, half the group scored between 13 and 17 points.

Inferential statistics determine whether observed differences among groups are significant or due to chance, and they allow you to draw conclusions about the population from which you sampled. That is, you may be able to generalize findings beyond your particular group. However, in order to use these statistics, certain assumptions must be met, such as selection of random assignment informants. This chapter will not cover inferential statistics. Someone with statistics expertise can assist in conducting analyses if the experimental design has produced data that meet the necessary assumptions.

Descriptive Analysis
_____

Frequency distributions show the number of people who selected a particular answer to a survey or test question, obtained a certain score, answered a question, etc. In the example shown below, the first column shows scores and the second column shows how many people received each score. For example, 4 individuals out of 25 scored a six.

Cumulative frequencies show the total number of people falling below or above a certain score. To calculate cumulative frequencies add all the frequencies of the previous scores to the current one. For example 5 people scored 5 points or lower on the test in the example below.

Percentages are calculated by dividing the number of individuals who obtained a particular score (or selected a certain response) by the total number who took the test (or answered the question) and multiplying by 100. The percentage of those scoring a 6 on this test is calculated in this way:

Step 1: 4÷25 = .16
Step 2: .16 x 100 = 16%

Example
_____

Score	Frequency	Cumulative Frequency	Percentage	Cumulative Percentage
0	0	0	0%	0%
1	0	0	0%	0%
2	0	0	0%	0%
3	1	1	4%	4%
4	2	3	8%	12%
5	2	5	8%	20%
6	4	9	16%	36%
7	6	15	24%	60%
8	5	20	20%	80%
9	3	23	12%	92%
10	2	25	8%	100%
N=	25	25	100%	100%

```
Number of                        X
 students                        X  X
obtaining                     X  X  X
    score                     X  X  X  X
                        X  X  X  X  X  X  X
                     X  X  X  X  X  X  X  X
                  0  1  2  3  4  5  6  7  8  9  10
                           Test Scores
```

Cumulative percentages are calculated in the same way as cumulative frequencies: add all the percentages of the previous scores to the current one. Sixty percent of those in the example given score 7 or lower. If you want to know the percentage of those who scored 7 or higher, subtract the percentage of those who scored less than 7 from 100: 100% - 36% = 64%.

The **mode** of a distribution is the score of a test (or answer to a question) that has the highest frequency. In the above example, the mode is 7.

The **median** is the point above and below which one-half of the scores are found. If the total number of those who took the test is even, the median is the number half way between the two middle scores. In the example, we can look at the cumulative frequency column and determine that the median is 7 since the 50th percentile lies within the score of 7.

The **mean** is the average. It is the sum of all the values divided by the number of values. In the example the scores of 25 respondents equals 174; 174÷25=7.

The **variance** is the extent to which all the values vary from the mean. To obtain the variance, the difference between each value and the mean for every subject is squared, and all such values are added. That number is then divided by the total number of subjects:

$$\frac{(3\text{-}7)^2 + (3\text{-}7)^2 + (4\text{-}7)^2 \ldots}{25} = 3.24$$

The **standard deviation** is the square root of the variance; in our case 1.8. If you represent a frequency distribution by its mean, also provide the standard deviation, which allows the reader to judge how representative the mean was for the subject population. An easy way to obtain the mean, variance, and standard deviation is by using a calculator. Calculators with statistical functions will provide the statistics after you have entered each value in the distribution. If you are planning to evaluate a community-wide effort, consider the use of a personal computer to analyze data.

Percentage change will tell you how much a program has improved program participants' knowledge by calculating the relative change from the pre-test to the post-test. This can be done for each individual and also for the group as a whole. Subtract the individual (or group mean) pre-test score from the post-test score and divide the resulting figure by the pre-test score. Our mean post-test score was 7. In this case, the score was the mean post-test score for a group of social service providers. If our mean pre-test score had been 5, then the percentage change would be:

    Step 1: 7 - 5 = 2
    Step 2: 2÷5=.4
    Step 3: .4 x 100 = 40%

*Summarizing
Open-ended
Questions*

Interviews and questionnaires often contain open-ended questions to which the respondent is not given a choice of answers, but must provide a response. Program feedback questions are often of this type. For example, an item on your evaluation form asks "What did you like best about the workshop?" You may get an idea of the participants' views by simply reading through the answers. However, there is a more systematic way of looking at the information you collect.

The first step in summarizing results to open-ended questions is to review a sample of the answers. From your review and prior experience with the question(s), construct response categories into which you will place individual answers. As you assign answers to these categories, you may find it necessary to change, combine, delete, or add categories. This is fine as long as you reassign any responses you classified before making the changes.

Be generous with the number of categories you create; it is easier to combine unnecessary categories after reviewing all the answers than it is to distinguish responses within categories. However, be sure that you can easily distinguish among categories when assigning answers. It is inevitable that you will encounter answers that don't quite fit your list of categories. Put these answers in an "Other" category, but try to minimize them. After categorizing all responses you can calculate the percentage of responses in each category.

Example

Example of Coding an Open-ended Question

Below is a list of hypothetical responses to the question, "What should two teenagers consider before they decide whether or not to become sexually active?" After reading the following answers, list the major categories that emerge from the responses.

- Are they really ready
- Do they really care for each other
- She might get pregnant
- They might get VD or AIDS
- Birth control
- Pregnant
- If she got pregnant what should they do
- Make sure that when it's time they're both ready

- Could they take care of a baby
- Should they tell their parents
- They really like each other
- Do they love each other
- She might get pregnant
- Do they have protection
- Do they have birth control

The following table shows one way to categorize the responses. The three leading considerations regarding sexual activity seem to be: the possibility of pregnancy, use of birth control, and the quality of the relationship.

Category	Frequency	Percent
A) Possibility of pregnancy:	5	33%
B) Use of birth control:	3	20%
C) Maturity:	2	13.%
D) Quality of relationship:	3	20%
E) Parents:	1	7%
F) STDs:	1	7%
	15	**100%**

Sometimes answers are difficult to classify. For example, "Are they really ready" could be thought of as belonging in either the maturity category or the quality of relationship category. The best way to check your judgment is to have a second staff person (or program volunteer) classify the same answers. There should be agreement on at least 8 out of 10 classifications, or an 80 percent inter-judge reliability score. If scores are lower, review the answers where there is disagreement and make sure your categories are appropriate. At this point, overlapping or insufficiently distinct categories can be combined; for example, maturity and quality of relationship may lend themselves to being combined, as they are often interrelated.

Preparing the Results for Presentation

Now that the data have been collected and analyzed, you will want to present it clearly to others. Tables and charts are often a good way to display information. However, they should always be accompanied by a narrative summary of the same results. One potential community-based intervention discussed earlier is the establishment of school-based health clinics that provide a variety of medical, health education, and mental health services to adolescents. One goal of such clinics is the prevention of unintended teen pregnancies. Below is a hypothetical example of year-end survey data of reported contraceptive use for those eleventh and twelfth grade students who report being sexually active. The results compare reported contraceptive use by students attending two schools — one with a school based clinic (school A) and one with no clinic (school B). Students were asked, "Did you use birth control (pill, condom, sponge) the last time you had sex?" "N" refers to the number of sexually active students who answered the question. Thus 350 students attending School A who were sexually active answered the question on birth control. A table such as the one below supplements discussion and helps clarify the evaluation results. This information is even more illuminating as it provides data for each school before the school clinic was instituted.

Example

Reported Use of Birth Control at Last Intercourse by School

	School A (clinic) (N=350)		School B (no clinic) (N=390)	
	Pre	*Post*	*Pre*	*Post*
Yes	45%	55%	40%	45%
No	55%	45%	60%	55%

As shown, students at both schools improved their overall use of contraceptives, although sexually active students at School B (without a clinic) were less likely to use contraceptives and demonstrated a smaller increase in their use.

Another way to present information is with the use of a chart. For example, suppose you have measured change in parents' behavioral intent with the following question:

"In the next two weeks how likely are you to talk with your teenager about sex or birth control?" The figure below illustrates participants' change in intent from pre-test to post-test after attending three communication skills workshops. The proportion stating that they were very likely to talk to their teen jumped from 65 percent on the pre-test to 80 percent on the post-test. In your narrative, you could also note that these results reflect a shift in responses from the "not sure" and "not very likely" categories to the "very likely" category. You could also discuss some factors that contributed to the changes.

Example chart

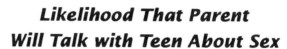

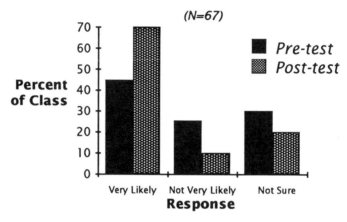

Your program results may not show this level of positive change. In that case, you still have the responsibility of presenting results and providing probable reasons why the expected results did not emerge.

Below is a line chart of birthrates for teenagers age 15-19 for an intervention and comparison county. Note that the intervention began in 1989 and initial results did not appear until 1991, demonstrating the value of continuing to collect data to be sure that one is able to document change over time.

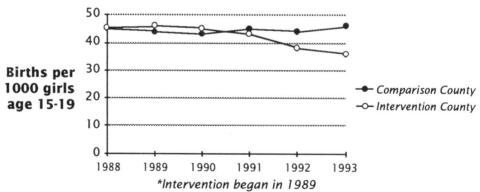

Step 10:
Report
Findings

Informing people of the evaluation findings is another step in making the evaluation count. It is certainly a requirement of any funding source, and it is also a way to contribute to the existing body of knowledge in the field of pregnancy prevention. You will want to prepare a report informing the funding sources, project staff, and other interested groups of the findings of the evaluation. You may find that sections of the evaluation can also help document and support the need for additional funding.

You do not have to wait until the evaluation is complete to begin preparing a report. In fact, it will be much easier to describe the study methods if you do not wait until you are finished. If you plan to disseminate the results, either in a newsletter or journal, you may want to present your evaluation in the report format outlined below. Before any information is disseminated, however, have your original community advisory board review and approve the working document.

*Components of
the Report*

a. **Summary:** State the goals and objectives of the community-wide effort and of individual programs, the methods of data collection, and the results of the evaluation. This short section gives the reader a concise picture of the program and its impact.

b. **Background:** Describe the history of the effort, your organizational structure, participating organizations, results of the needs assessment, target population(s), length of the program, significant activities, and parts of the program that are unique.

c. **Description of the Evaluation Study:** Describe the design, method(s) of data collection, sampling procedures, and the rationale. Describe any limitations that were encountered and how they were resolved.

d. **Results of the Study:** In this section, present the findings of the study without much interpretation. For example, show attendance counts, statistical analyses of data, and comparisons between groups. The program may also produce unintended or unanticipated consequences. These can be either positive or negative. For example, as a result of one family communication program, former participants developed a group that advocates for family life education programs which bring parents and children together to discuss family values. This unexpected result demonstrated support of the program. Be sure to include informal findings such as these. Sometimes quotes by program participants or anecdotes help make a report more memorable.

e. **Discussion of Results:** Provide interpretation and explanation of findings. Even if the findings are not what had been originally expected, insights from the program may help the next person (or group) who plans a program for a similarly targeted population.

f. **Conclusions and Recommendations:** Briefly summarize findings. Make recommendations based on the findings, such as necessary revisions in objectives, changes in curriculum, expansion of the program, and policy changes.

Step 11: Act on Findings

The ultimate purpose of an evaluation is to provide a basis for decisions. You want to find out how well the program is meeting its objectives and how it can be improved. As evaluations require a significant commitment of resources and staff, the results should be made as useful as possible for program management and personnel. If the evaluation demonstrates that the program was extremely effective or produced some unanticipated beneficial results, let people know about it. An evaluation can be an impressive way to build community support for the project. If, on the other hand, the evaluation uncovered program areas in need of revision, work on solving those problems so that the next evaluation will show greater progress in meeting stated objectives.

Listed below are ways that the program can use evaluation results:

Program Feedback and Improvement

- Assessing the quality of services the program has delivered.

- Modifying program materials and topics to better suit participant needs.

- Helping participants assess their own knowledge base.

- Preparing participants for future sessions.

- Increasing staff morale.

Assessing Impact of Program

- Determining the impact of the content and the effectiveness of the method(s) used in the program.

- Determining the perceived usefulness of the program for the target population(s).

Program Planning

- Planning for future programs based on the knowledge of what is most effective.

- Assessing community needs on an ongoing basis and planning programs to address those needs.

- Presenting results to funders for expansion of programs and establishment of potential private and public funding partnerships.

Complying with Program Requirements

- Completing quarterly and annual reports documenting how program objectives are being met.

- Presenting the results of the efforts to different policy makers, including the coalition's board of directors and local legislators.

Additionally, as program funds become more scarce, important decisions need to be made about where resources will be allocated. It is important to base these decisions on evidence of the impact of programs. It is just as important to learn what works as what does not work, so that we can develop the most effective programs for our communities. Evaluation results can be effective tools to document how our work is producing changes. Evaluation is also a way to provide evidence that we can respond to community needs as they undergo major shifts or changes.

Summary

The role of evaluation cannot be over-emphasized in our guide to community-wide adolescent pregnancy prevention initiatives. Unless the coalition has developed and built into its plan an evaluation component, it will have little or no ability to assess the effectiveness of its activities, and it will have no reliable capacity to determine what is working and what requires revision. It will also have little in the way of meaningful information to support requests for renewed and additional funding. Furthermore, there will be a critical lack of material needed to publicize the effectiveness and value of the coalition's activities. Clearly, without proper evaluation the coalition's programs will not possess a great capacity for survival.

Including case examples and an outline of the eleven steps in the evaluation process has made this our longest and most detailed chapter. However, if the coalition's efforts have been well thought out, and the planning and implementation steps have been thorough, the evaluation process can become a fulfilling and verifying experience that can lead to more effective action within the community, and also assist other groups nationwide in their efforts to address the problems associated with teenage pregnancy.

Appendix 8-1

Using a Random Numbers Table

Suppose that you want to sample 50 people out of a population of 200. To begin, arrange the population in a list. It is not necessary to number each item if you can count down the list. Next determine the number of digits you will need to use in the random number you select. Because our population is 200 we will be working with 3 digits. Look at the table on the next page; it represents a series of random numbers in the range from 00001 to 99999.

You must now make several decisions:

1. To read the table vertically or horizontally;

2. Where to start;

3. To look at the first 3 or last 3 digits of each 5 digit number.

It doesn't matter how you answer these questions as long as you stick with your decision while selecting the entire sample. Let's move vertically through the table, starting with the upper left number, and look only at the 3 left-most digits. The first number we will look at is 07092. Since we decided to look at the 3 left digits the first person in our sample will be the 70th person on our list. The next number moving down the column is 463. But there are only 200 persons on our list. How can we pick number 463? We don't. Skip that number and continue on until you come to a number that is 200 or less. In this case the second person to be selected in our sample will be the 117th person on our list, because the next number we can use is 11742. Continue in this fashion until you have selected 50 people.

What if you wanted to do a telephone survey of your city? The local telephone directory will be your list of the population from which to sample. One strategy would be to count how many entries are in the book and count down through the pages every time you have a random number. However this is too time consuming and laborious. Another way is to randomly select a page in the directory, then a column, and finally an entry in the column. You would need to repeat this procedure for each person in your sample.

07092	54592	24623	12067	06558	40944
46301	04181	44866	08306	25555	16148
61570	03660	06133	66735	66148	95145
31625	83799	01679	18941	31569	76448
93612	61718	99355	60870	94251	25841
11742	69681	44369	30827	62797	36118
43661	28859	10116	45645	93049	04499
96086	20748	38286	04491	55751	18962
49540	13181	08429	84183	69098	29661
36786	26366	37948	21569	41959	86660
09243	44204	86261	03167	30269	75356
97956	35018	40894	88629	25450	82251
93762	59530	46781	98885	56631	68626
27621	11225	04922	86264	65666	59434
60120	64418	40971	20394	95917	63866
45156	54859	01837	25996	76249	70886
05545	55043	01097	46508	09611	83744
14871	60650	32404	66245	50451	04322
68976	74951	94051	75089	78085	09194
57048	86256	27795	93692	09259	56546
97869	85344	63055	91718	45643	54144
89160	97192	22425	09663	35055	45489
25966	88220	62871	39265	02845	25862
81443	31719	05049	54086	34609	07563
11322	51931	44562	34386	08624	97863

General Resource Directory

---

*A*s your community develops its individual plan, a variety of specific programmatic questions will need answers. We encourage you to learn from and build upon the experience of others in the field and to call upon them for aid in determining what programs to develop and integrate in your own community. This directory includes organizations that are concerned with adolescent pregnancy prevention and related issues, including AIDS and other sexually-transmitted diseases, adolescent male involvement in teen pregnancy, school-based health clinics, family life education, funding, and contraception. In addition, a topical bibliography of books, manuals, and other publications which are relevant to the field follows. These resources may provide valuable assistance to service providers and others in establishing, implementing, and evaluating programs, but should not be considered an exhaustive listing as there are numerous helpful agencies in many regions throughout the country, as well as a multitude of worthwhile books and publications in the field of adolescent pregnancy and pregnancy prevention.

Organizations

Academy for Educational Development
100 Fifth Avenue
New York, NY 10010
(212) 243-1110

The AED addresses educational, social, health and cultural issues with a variety of projects. Currently, the AED is involved with middle schools and community agencies in adolescent pregnancy prevention efforts in school districts nationwide. In addition, their Support Center for Educational Equity, which focuses primarily on educational opportunities for parenting teens, maintains a variety of resources on adolescent pregnancy prevention efforts.

The Alan Guttmacher Institute

2010 Massachusetts Avenue NW   111 Fifth Avenue
Washington, D.C. 20036   New York, NY 10003
(202) 296-4012   (212) 254-5656

AGI works to develop adequate family planning and sex education programs through policy analysis, public education, and research. The Institute publishes extensively, including many research reports regarding adolescent pregnancy and prevention, such as *Factbook on Teenage Pregnancy*, and *Teenage Pregnancy in the United States, the Scope of the Problem and State Responses*. AGI publishes the journal, *Family Planning Perspectives*, which includes many articles of interest to those working in adolescent pregnancy prevention.

American Civil Liberties Union (ACLU)

132 W. 43rd Street
New York, NY 10036
(212) 944-9800

The ACLU champions the rights set forth in the Declaration of Independence and the U.S. Constitution, as well as the right to a safe and legal abortion for all women. It publishes a monthly newsletter, *First Principles*, and a bimonthly newspaper, *Civil Liberties*. The ACLU has branches throughout the country which work with different groups to ensure access to reproductive health care for minors.

Center for Early Adolescence

Suite 223, Car Mill Mall
Carrboro, NC 27510
(919) 966-1148

As part of the Department of Maternal and Child Health at the University of North Carolina at Chapel Hill, the Center disseminates information such as resource lists and bibliographies that deal with school-age children and adolescents. The center's quarterly newsletter is filled with valuable resources such as programs, research, books, films, and conferences for professionals who work with teenagers.

Center for Population Options

1025 Vermont Avenue NW
Washington, D.C. 20005
(202) 347-5700

CPO works to enhance opportunities in key decision-making areas of adolescents' lives: continuing their education, planning their families, and obtaining needed health and social services, with a focus on preventing too-early childbearing. CPO publishes three quarterlies: *Options, Clinic News,* and *Passages* (in three languages for international audiences). An important part of CPO is its Support Center for School-based Clinics, which provides individual technical assistance, regional training, an annual conference, publications, and a quarterly newsletter on program and policy developments. Other key areas of concern include life-planning education, HIV/AIDS prevention, and developing peer programs. CPO's *Publications List* details its resources.

The CPO has also developed a hands-on advocacy training workshop called "Controversy" for people who are not experienced advocates. The training was designed for people who work primarily as administrators or community service providers in areas concerning adolescent pregnancy, adolescent reproductive health care, and/or family planning. The workshop takes a minimum of 2 1/2 hours and is in two parts: 1) An introduction to community advocacy, and 2) a role-play game that allows participants to practice advocacy skills. For more information, write or call Rebecca Stone, Center for Population Options, 1012 14th Street N.W., Suite 1200, Washington, D.C., 20005. (202) 347-5700.

Center for Reproductive Health Policy Research
University of California San Francisco
1388 Sutter Street, 11th Floor
San Francisco, CA 94109
(415) 476-5254

Within the Institute for Health Policy Studies, the Center represents a collaborative effort of the Department of Obstetrics, Gynecology and Reproductive Sciences, School of Medicine, UCSF, and the School of Public Health, UC Berkeley. Emphasis is on analysis of state and federal policies affecting the provision of reproductive health services in the areas of family planning cost effectiveness, sexually transmitted diseases, adolescent pregnancy and pregnancy prevention, and the family planning needs of special population groups. In addition, the Center focuses on the evaluation of service programs, including school-based health centers and comprehensive prenatal and maternal care.

Children's Defense Fund
122 C Street NW
Washington, D.C. 20001
(202) 628-8787

This organization is a national children's advocacy group working for changes in policies and programs which affect the rights of children. CDF's goal is to educate the nation about the needs of children and encourage preventive investment in children before troubles arise. Its Adolescent Pregnancy Prevention Clearinghouse publishes six reports per year on America's teenage pregnancy crisis and its solutions; some important reports have included: "Model Programs: Preventing Adolescent Pregnancy and Building Youth Self-Sufficiency," "Preventing Children Having Children," and "Preventing Adolescent Pregnancy: What Schools Can Do." For more information, write to "Publications" at the above address. In addition, CDF sponsors an annual conference which provides valuable information on adolescent pregnancy.

Child Welfare League of America
440 1st Street NW
Washington, D.C. 20001
(202) 638-2952

This is an advocacy organization which works on numerous child welfare issues, including several related to adolescent pregnancy. The organization sponsors an annual conference which includes sessions on adolescent pregnancy prevention, in addition to other child-related issues.

ETR Associates (Education, Training, Research)
P.O. Box 1830
Santa Cruz, CA 95061-1830
(408) 438-4060

ETR Associates is a private, non-profit family life and health education organization serving health care providers, teachers, and other professionals from schools, health organizations, community education, and youth-serving agencies nationwide. Its services include: offering training and technical assistance in basic health education preparation; development and evaluation of educational approaches; and collecting and disseminating materials and data on family life education, AIDS, adolescent pregnancy prevention, and risk-taking behaviors of young people. In addition, Network Publications, a division of ETR Associates, is the country's largest publisher of family life and health education resources, publishing and distributing numerous videos, guides, books, pamphlets, workbooks, and two quarterly magazines: *Family Life Educator* and the *California AIDS Clearinghouse Reviewer*.

Family Resource Coalition
230 North Michigan Avenue
Suite 1625
Chicago, IL 60601
(312) 726-4750

A membership network for organizations interested in family and parenting issues which attempts to improve the content and expand the number of available programs. Teenage parenthood prevention is a special focus of this group.

Girls Clubs of America
205 Lexington Avenue
New York, NY 10016
(212) 689-3700

This national group has developed and conducts a four-part adolescent pregnancy program which includes "Growing Together," for 9-12 year-old girls; "Will Power—Won't Power," for 12-14 year-old girls; and "Choices and Career Awareness" and

"Health Bridge" for 15-18 year-old girls. These programs are currently being implemented in approximately 50 Girls Clubs nationwide.

National Abortion Federation
900 Pennsylvania Avenue SE
Washington, D.C. 20003
(202) 546-9060

The Federation is a political action group dedicated to sustaining a pro-choice political constituency in order to maintain the right to a legal abortion for all women. It publishes the NARAL *Newsletter* quarterly.

National Board of the YWCA
726 Broadway
New York, NY 10003
(212) 614-2700

The YWCA is implementing a variety of teen pregnancy/parenting programs throughout the country, including several prevention programs using media.

National Center for Youth Law
1663 Mission Street
San Francisco, CA 94103
(415) 543-3307

The National Center for Youth Law is a non-profit organization devoted to improving the lives of poor children in the United States. NCYL attorneys are experts in the various areas of law that affect children, including child and adolescent health, emancipation of minors, juvenile justice and court procedures, and public benefit programs for children. These attorneys are available to assist advocates in a variety of ways, including discussing particular cases, researching legal issues, conducting training programs and materials, and lending written materials from their library.

National Conference of State Legislatures
1050 17th Street, Suite 2100
Denver, CO 80265
(303) 623-7800

The Children, Youth and Families Program of the National Conference of State Legislatures is designed to meet the needs of state legislatures in developing policy and programs related to children and families. Project areas include Child Care, Child Support Enforcement and Child Welfare, in addition to their Teen Pregnancy Project. The Teen Pregnancy Project responds to requests from legislative staff with information and resources about topics that include family life education, school-based health clinics, contraception, abortion and related issues, and outreach to young males.

National Family Planning and Reproductive Health Association, Inc.
122 C Street Suite 380
Washington, D.C. 20001
(202) 628-3535

This association works to improve family planning and reproductive health services by acting as a national communication network. It publishes the *NFPRHA News & Report* monthly as well as various papers, and conducts an annual conference for service providers and others concerned with maintaining family planning services throughout the country.

National Organization on Adolescent Pregnancy and Parenting, Inc.
Washington D.C. Area Office
P.O. Box 2365
Reston, VA 22090
(703) 435-3948

This is a national membership network dedicated to preventing adolescent pregnancy and problems related to adolescent sexuality, pregnancy and parenting. It provides in-depth membership newsletters, and sponsors an annual conference and other training for professionals concerned with adolescent pregnancy and parenting adolescents.

National Resource Center for Youth Services
University of Oklahoma
125 No. Greenwood Avenue
Tulsa, OK 74120
(918) 585-2986

The resource center's *Partnerships for Youth 2000: A Program Models Manual* describes 72 community-level programs which are effectively addressing the problems identified by the Youth 2000 Initiative—illiteracy, school dropouts, alcohol and other substance abuse, unemployment, teen pregnancy, and others.

National Urban League, Inc.
500 E. 62nd Street
New York, NY 10021
(212) 310-9000

The Urban League works nationally to ensure equal opportunities for socially and economically disadvantaged persons. It currently conducts three national programs addressing adolescent pregnancy and parenting, including the Adolescent Male Responsibility Project, which is a public awareness campaign to encourage responsible male involvement in pregnancy prevention and parenting.

Office of Adolescent Pregnancy Programs

HHS Bldg. Rm 733-E

200 Independence Avenue SW

Washington, D.C. 20201

(202) 245-7473

This is a Department of Health and Human Services Agency which funds and supervises federal programs related to adolescent pregnancy prevention and parenting throughout the country.

Planned Parenthood Federation of America

810 7th Avenue

New York, NY 10019

(212) 541-7800

Planned Parenthood has a long-term and well-documented commitment to the reduction of adolescent pregnancy and childbearing, which is embodied in its mission statement, services, and activities. PPFA provides informative, educational and contraceptive counseling and services through a nationwide system of clinics, and also collaborates with numerous other organizations in achieving its goals. The organization also publishes extensively in the field of adolescent pregnancy prevention. In addition, PPFA provides a valuable library service, the Library and Information Network (LINK), which publishes bibliographies of resources on numerous topics. For more information, write to the Department of Education at the above address.

Search Institute

122 W. Franklin Avenue, Suite 525

Minneapolis, MN 55404

(612) 870-9511

The Institute is a research organization which provides information on programs about adolescents and family life to social service professionals. Its programs encourage traditional family and sexual values. It publishes a sex education curriculum for junior high school students and their parents, *Human Sexuality: Values and Choices.*

Sex Information and Education Council of the U.S.

80 5th Avenue Suite 801

New York, NY 10011

(212) 929-2300

SIECUS is one of the largest national clearinghouses for information on sexuality. In addition to publishing sex education curricula, SIECUS also publishes newsletters, books and reports.

Social Research Applications
170 State Street, Suite 280
Los Altos, CA 94022
(415) 949-3487

This agency specializes in furthering scientifically valid projects on social interventions, especially in the area of teenage pregnancy prevention. It is involved with encouraging more scientific evaluations on the impact of teenage pregnancy upon society.

Sociometrics
170 State Street, Suite 260
Los Altos, CA 94022
(415) 949-3282

Sociometrics is a social science archive devoted to intervention research in a variety of areas. Their "Data Archives on Adolescent Pregnancy & Pregnancy Prevention" (DAAPPP) contain not only research and development in the field but over 150 sets of computerized data dealing with teenage pregnancy, which are available at cost.

Topical Bibliography

Abortion

Emmens, C. *The Abortion Controversy*. 1987. Julian Messner & Simon Schuster, Inc. New York, NY.

Melton, G.B. & Pliner, A.J. *Adolescent Abortion: Psychological and Legal Issues*. 1986. University of Nebraska Press. Lincoln, NE.

Sheeran, P. *Women, Society, the State: Abortion*. 1987. Greenwood Press, Inc. Westport, CT.

Adolescent Males and Teen Pregnancy

Beckstein, D. "1986: An Annotated Guide to Men's Sexuality and Reproductive Health." 1986. EPA. Campbell, CA.

Bingham, M., Quinn, L. & Sheehan, W. *Challenges: A Young Man's Journal for Self-Awareness & Personal Planning*. 1988. Advocacy Press. Santa Barbara, CA.

Dryfoos, J. *Putting the Boys in the Picture: A Review of Programs to Promote Sexual Responsibility Among Young Males*. 1988. Network Publications, ETR Associates, Santa Cruz, CA.

Robinson, B. *Teenage Fathers*. 1988. D.C. Heath and Company. Lexington, MA.

Adolescent Pregnancy
———————

Adolescent Pregnancy Childwatch Manual, available through the Children's Defense Fund, 122 C Street, Washington, D.C., 20001. This guide includes information on how to conduct community surveys and interviews (primarily conducted by volunteers) to determine the maternal and child health needs of the local population.

Adolescent Parenthood: Developing a Comprehensive Community Planning Guide Around the Issue of Teenage Pregnancy, and *Adolescent Parenthood: Developing a State Plan Around the Issue of Teenage Pregnancy*, both edited by Anita Mitchell for Women and Foundations/Corporate Philanthropy, 141 Fifth Avenue, New York, NY, 10010. These two planning manuals are helpful in organizing a planning conference on adolescent pregnancy during the early stages of community development.

Adolescent Pregnancy Prevention
———————

Barth, R.P. *Reducing the Risk: Building Skills to Prevent Pregnancy*. 1989. Garland Publishing, Inc. New York, NY.

Bingham, M., Quinn, L. & Sheehan, W. *Mother Daughter Choices: A Handbook for the Coordinator*. 1988. Advocacy Press. Santa Barbara, CA.

Johnson, J. et al. "First Things First." 1989. Planned Parenthood of New York. New York, NY.

Lindsay, J. & Rodine, S. *Teen Pregnancy Challenge: Strategies for Change*. 1989. Morning Glory Press. Buena Vista, CA.

Lindsay, J. & Rodine, S. *Teen Pregnancy Challenge: Programs for Kids*. 1989. Morning Glory Press. Buena Vista, CA.

Peterson, L. "Helping Teens Wait." 1987. The Center for Health Training. Seattle, WA.

AIDS and Sexually Transmitted Diseases
———————

Brick, P. et al. *Teaching Safer Sex*. 1989. Planned Parenthood of Bergen County, Inc., NJ.

Quackenbush, M., Nelson, M., & Clark, K., eds. *The AIDS Challenge: Prevention Education for Young People*. 1988. Network Publications, ETR Associates. Santa Cruz, CA.

Quackenbush, M. & Sargent, P. *Teaching AIDS—A Resource Guide on Acquired Immune Deficiency Syndrome*. 1988. Network Publications, ETR Associates. Santa Cruz, CA.

Stensrud, A. *Breaking the Chain: A Sexually Transmitted Disease Teaching Guide*. 1986. Planned Parenthood of St. Louis, MO.

Tseng, C. H., Villanueva, T. G., & Powell, A. *Sexually Transmitted Diseases: A Handbook.* 1987. R & E Publishers, CA.

Controversial Issues

Bender, D. & Leone, B. *Teenage Sexuality: Opposing Viewpoints.* 1988. Greenhaven Press. St. Paul, MN.

Network Publications. *Beyond Reproduction: Tips and Techniques for Teaching Sensitive Family Life Education Issues.* 1983. Network Publications, ETR Associates, Santa Cruz, CA.

Development and Evaluation of Programs

Brindis, C. & Reyes, P. *Evaluating Your Information and Education Project.* 1988. Center for Population and Reproductive Health Policy, University of California, San Francisco, CA., EPA, Campbell CA.

Brindis, C., Korenbrot, C. & Brown, P. *Evaluation Guidebook for Family Planning Information and Education Projects.* 1986. EPA, Campbell, CA.

Card, J. J., Editor. *Evaluating Programs Aimed at Preventing Teenage Pregnancies.* 1989. Sociometrics Corporation. Los Altos, CA.

Center for Dropout Prevention. *What Works and Why: A Guide to Evaluating Teen Pregnancy/Parenting Programs.* 1988. University of Miami Press. Coral Gables, FL.

Davis, C., Yarber, W., & Davis, S. *Sexuality-Related Measures: A Compendium.* 1988. Graphic Publishing Company. Lake Mills, IA.

Herman, J. *Program Evaluation Kit,* 2nd Ed. 1988. Sage Publications. Newbury Park, CA.

Johnson, K. & Rosenbaum, S. "Building Health Programs for Teenagers: Clearinghouse Paper No. 4." 1986. Children's Defense Fund. Washington, D.C.

Philliber, S. "Evaluating Your Adolescent Pregnancy Program: How To Get Started." 1989. Children's Defense Fund, Adolescent Pregnancy Prevention Clearinghouse. Washington, D.C.

Rossi, P. & Freeman, H. *Evaluation: A Systematic Approach.* 1985. Sage Publications. Newbury Park, CA.

Treanor, B. *Barriers in Developing Comprehensive and Effective Youth Services.* 1989. American Youth Work Center. Washington, D.C.

Zabin, L. S. & Hirsch, M.B. *Evaluation of Pregnancy Programs in the School Context.* 1988. Lexington Books. Lexington, MA.

Family Life
Education

Abbey, N. *Family Life Education: Homework for Parents and Teens.* 1984. Network Publications, ETR Associates, Santa Cruz, CA.

The Alan Guttmacher Institute. *Risk and Responsibility: Teaching Sex Education in America's Schools Today.* 1989. The Alan Guttmacher Institute. New York, NY.

Alter, J., Cook, A.T., & Wilson, P. "Teaching Parents to be the Primary Sexuality Educators of Their Children, Volume II: Guide to Designing and Implementing Multisession Courses." 1982. Mathtech, Inc. Bethesda, MD.

Cassell, C. & Wilson, P. *Sexuality Education: A Resource Book.* 1989. Garland Publishing, Inc. New York, NY.

Compton, N., Duncan, M., & Hruska, J. *How Schools Can Combat Student Pregnancy.* 1987. NEA Professional Library. West Haven, CT.

Gasiorowski, J. *Adolescent Sexuality and Sex Education: A Handbook for Parents and Educators.* 1988. Wm. C. Brown Co. IA.

Hamrick, M. "Sexuality Knowledge Test for Early Adolescents (Ages 10-14)." Spring, 1988. *Family Life Educator.* Network Publications, ETR Associates, Santa Cruz, CA.

Search Institute. *Values & Choices.* 1987. Search Institute, MN.

Vincent, M.L. *Reducing Unintended Adolescent Pregnancy Through School/Community Educational Interventions: A South Carolina Case Study.* 1988. Centers for Disease Control. Atlanta, GA.

Weikart, D. et al. "Changed Lives: The Effects of the Perry Preschool Program on Youths Through Age 19." 1984. The High/Scope Press. Ypsilanti, MI.

Wilson, S. *Creating Family Life Education Programs in the Public Schools: A Guide for State Education Policymakers.* 1985. National Association of State Boards of Education. Alexandria, VA.

Family Planning

Hatcher, R., Guest, F., Stewart, F., Stewart, G., Trussell, J., Bowen, S., & Cates, W. *Contraceptive Technology.* 1988-1989. Printed Matter Inc. Atlanta, GA.

Spain, J. *Sexual, Contraceptive and Pregnancy Choices: Counseling Adolescents.* 1988. Printed Matter, Inc. Atlanta, GA.

Funding

Adamson. T. A. *Inside Grant & Project Writing: How to Write Projects That Get Funded.* 1979. Pam Publishers. Salinas, CA.

Ashton, D. *The Complete Guide to Planned Giving: Everything You Need to Know to Compete Successfully for Major Gifts.* 1988. JLA Publication. Cambridge, MA.

Bauer, D. *The How-To Grants Manual: Successful Grant-seeking Techniques for Obtaining Public/Private Grants.* 1988. The American Council on Education. New York, NY.

Renz, L., Ed. *The Foundation Directory.* 1985. The Foundation Center. New York, NY.

English, A. & Tereskowitz, L. *School-Based Health Clinics: Legal Issues.* 1988. National Center for Youth Law & Center for Population Options. San Francisco, CA.

Gilman, S. & Nader, P. "Measuring the Effectiveness of a School Health Program: Methods and Preliminary Analysis." 1982. *Journal of School Health* 49(1).

Hadley, E., Kirby, D. & Lovick, S. *School-based Health Clinics: A Guide to Implementing Programs.* 1986. Support Center for School-Based Clinics/Center for Population Options. Washington, D.C.

Iverson, D. "Promoting Health Through the Schools: A Challenge for the Eighties." 1981. *Health Education Quarterly* 8(1).

Kirby, D. & Waszak, C. "School-Based Clinics Enter the '90s: Update, Evaluation and Future Challenges." 1989. Center for Population Options. Washington, D.C.

Newman, I. "Integrating Health Services and Health Education: Seeking a Balance." *Journal of School Health,* October, 1982.

Newman, I. & Newman, E. "School Health Services, Health Education and the School Environment: Do They Fit Together?" *Journal of School Health,* March, 1980.

Oda, D., DeAngelis, C., Berman, B., & Meeker, B. "The Resolution of Health Problems in School Children." *Journal of School Health,* March, 1985.

School-based Clinics Support Center. "School-based Clinics: A Guide for Advocates." 1988. Publications Department, Center for Population Options. Washington, D.C.

Warren, C. *Improving Students' Access to Health Care: School-Based Health Clinics, A Briefing Paper for Policymakers.* 1987. Center for Public Advocacy Research, Inc. New York, NY.

School-based
Health Clinics

Additional Resources

American Home Economic Association
Accounting Office/Publication Sales
2010 Massachusetts Avenue NW
Washington, D.C. 20036-1028

Educating Adolescents About AIDS is an annotated list of materials to help teach teens about AIDS. It lists 45 resources including curricula, posters, films, videos, brochures, books, bibliographies and hotlines, and is available for $3.50 by writing the above address.

Current Literature in Family Planning
Department of Education, PPFA
810 Seventh Avenue
New York, NY 10019
(212) 541-7800

Monthly classified list of books and articles recently received in the Katherine Dexter Library in the field of family planning in the U.S.A. Book reviews as well as reviews of articles and subject bibliographies are included in the monthly review. Many of the subjects included are relevant to the field of adolescent pregnancy prevention, including STDs, teenagers and sexuality, and clinic services.

Family Life Information Exchange
P.O. Box 10716
Rockville, MD 20850
(301) 770-3662

This is a clearinghouse for information on family planning, adolescent pregnancy and adoption. Upon request, the exchange will provide a listing of publications, posters and bibliographies which can be obtained free of charge.

Family Resources Database
National Council on Family Relations
1910 West County Road B
Suite 147
St. Paul, MN 55113

A computerized core collection of literature, programs, directories and services for the family, and allied fields. Teenage pregnancy is one of its 130 subject areas.

Health Promotion Resource Center
Stanford Center for Research in Disease Prevention
1000 Welch Road
Palo Alto, CA 94304
(415) 723-0003

This group publishes manuals such as the present volume in addition to brief "How To" guides and other materials for those in the field of community-based health promotion. Write or telephone for a free catalog.

LINK (Library and Information Network) PPFA

810 Seventh Avenue
New York, NY 10019
(212) 541-7800

This library service provides valuable resource lists on many facets of family planning, including education, in the form of bibliographies. The service also publishes the journal, *Emphasis,* which highlights people and programs in the field of sexuality and population education. Please write for further information.

Public Affair Pamphlets

381 Park Avenue South
New York, NY 10016

Schools and Sex Education: New Perspectives is the title of a pamphlet published by this group presenting an overview and an update of the issues surrounding sex education in schools. It can be obtained for $1.00 by writing to the above address.

SHARE Resource Center on Teen Pregnancy Prevention

P.O. Box 30666
Bethesda, MD 20814
(301) 907-6523

This clearinghouse for data and information related to teen pregnancy prevention is available to program professionals as well as the general public. Database includes current materials on all programs, statistics and curricula from DHHS research and grants; similar information from the state and local level; and materials from the private sector.

Too-Early Childbearing Network

SWRL
4665 Lampson Avenue
Los Alamitos, CA 90720

This newsletter, funded by the Charles Stewart Mott Foundation, reports on programs, research findings and innovative ideas in the fields of adolescent pregnancy, prevention, and parenting issues.

Bibliography

Adams-Taylor, S. Morich, M., Pittman, K., and Adams, G. "What About the Boys? Teenage Pregnancy Prevention Strategies." *Adolescent Pregnancy Prevention Clearinghouse Report Series* (July/August). Washington, DC: The Children's Defense Fund, 1988.

Babbie, E. *The Practice of Social Research.* Belmont, CA: Wadsworth Publishing Company, 1983.

Brindis, C. and Jeremy, R. *Adolescent Pregnancy and Parenting in California: A Strategic Plan for Action.* San Francisco: Center for Reproductive Health Policy Research, University of California, San Francisco, 1988.

Brindis C., Korenbrot C., and Brown P. *Evaluation Guidebook for Family Planning Information and Education Projects.* State of California, Department of Health Services, Office of Family Planning, Grant #85-86970, 1986.

Brindis, C. and Reyes, P. *Evaluating your Information and Education Project*, California Department of Health Services, Distributed by Education Program Associates, Campbell, CA, 1988.

Brinkerhoff, R., Brethower, D., Hluchyj, T., and Nowakowski, J. *Program Evaluation: A Practitioner's Guide for Trainers and Educators* (Sourcebook/Casebook and Design Manual). Boston, MA: Kluwer-Nijhoff Publishing, 1983.

Brown, C. *The Art of Coalition Building: A Guide for Community Leaders*, American Jewish Committee, New York, NY, 1981.

Burghardt, S. *Organizing for Community Action.* Beverly Hills, CA: Sage Human Services Guide 27, 1982.

California Congress of Parents, Teachers, and Students, Inc. and the California State Department of Education. *A Guide to School and Community Action,* Sacramento, CA, 1981.

Campbell, D. and Stanley, J. *Experimental and Quasi-Experimental Designs for Research.* Chicago, IL: Rand McNally College Publishing Company, 1963.

Card, J. and Reagan, T. *Sourcebook of Comparison Data.* Los Altos, CA: Sociometrics Corporation, 1989.

Childwatch Manual, Children's Defense Fund, Washington, DC, 1987.

Community Council of Greater Dallas, *Impact 88: A Cumulative Report to the Community,* Dallas, TX, September, 1987.

Dawson, D. "The Effects of Sex Education on Adolescent Behavior." *Family Planning Perspectives* 18:162-170, 1986.

Dryfoos, J. *Adolescent-at-Risk: Prevalence and Prevention.* New York: Oxford Press, 1990.

Dunkle, M. and Nash, M. "Creating Effective Interagency Collaboratives." *Education Week*, March 15, 1989.

Forrest, J. and Silverman, J. "What Public School Teachers Teach About Preventing Pregnancy, AIDS, and Sexually Transmitted Diseases," *Family Planning Perspectives* 21:65-72, 1989.

Forrest, J. *Exploration of the Effects of Organized Family Planning Programs in the United States on Adolescent Fertility.* Final Report. Washington, DC: Alan Guttmacher Institute, 1980.

Hadley, E., Lovick, S., and Kirby, D. *School-Based Health Clinics: A Guide to Implementing Programs*, Washington, DC: Center for Population Options, October, 1986.

Hayes, C. (ed.). *Risking the Future: Adolescent Sexuality, Pregnancy, and Childbearing.* Washington, DC: National Academy Press, 1987.

Heimovics, R. and Kitzi, G. *Developing Alternative Solutions- The Nominal Group Process*, Unpublished Training Materials, Adolescent Resources Corporation, 4010 Washington, Suite 400, Kansas City, MO 64111, 1986.

Kenny, A., Guardado, S. and Brown, L. "Sex Education and AIDS Education in the Schools: What States and Large School Districts are Doing." *Family Planning Perspectives* 21:56-64, 1989.

Kimmich, M. "Addressing the Problem of Adolescent Pregnancy: The State of the Art and the Art in the States." Unpublished report, National Governors Association, November, 1985.

Kirby, D. "Sexuality Education: An Evaluation of Programs and their Effects – An Executive Summary." Santa Cruz, CA: Network Publications, 1984.

Kirby, D. and Waszah, C. "An Assessment of Six School-Based Clinics: Services, Impact, and Potential." Washington, DC: Center for Population Options, 1989.

Kiritz, N. *Program Planning and Proposal Writing,* New York: The Grantsmanship Center, Reprint Series on Program Planning and Proposal Writing, 1980,

Kisker, E. "Clinic Effectiveness in Serving Adolescents." *Family Planning Perspectives* 11:215-222, 1979.

Kitzi, G. *Community-Development.* Unpublished Training Materials, Adolescent Resources Corporation, 4010 Washington, Suite 400, Kansas City, MO 64111, 1986.

Kohn, S. and Maloney, P. "A Center for Change. Conflict and Challenge-Teen Programs Today. Planned Parenthood Federation of America." *Emphasis,* p. 4-5, Winter, 1985-86.

Koshel, J. *An Overview of State Policies Affecting Adolescent Pregnancy and Parenting.* Preliminary Report for the Carnegie Corporation, New York, NY, 1989.

Louis Harris and Associates, Inc. *American Teens Speak: Sex, Myth, T.V., and Birth Control.* New York, 1986.

Louis Harris and Associates, Inc. *Public Attitudes Toward Teenage Pregnancy, Sex, Education and Birth Control.* New York, 1988.

Marsiglio, W. and Mott, F. "The Impact of Sex Education on Sexual Activity, Contraceptive Use and Premarital Pregnancy Among American Teenagers." *Family Planning Perspectives* 18:151-162, 1986.

Nash, M. and Dunkle, M., *Promoting Collaboration, Promoting Success: Educators Working With Communities on Teenage Pregnancy and Parenting,* a publication of the Equity Center, 220 Eye Street, N.E., Suite 250, Washington, DC, 20002, 1988.

Ooms, T. and Herendeen, S. *The Unique Health Needs of Adolescents: Implications for Health Care Insurance and Financing.* A background briefing report and meeting highlights developed for the Family Impact Seminar, sponsored by the American Association for Marriage and Family Therapy, Research, and Education Foundation, Washington, DC, 1988.

Planned Parenthood Federation of America. *Community-Based Family Life Education.* LINK Reference Sheet 4, 1983.

Planned Parenthood of East Central Georgia, *Teen Pregnancy Prevention Programs for Rural America — A Study of an Approach the Works.* Unpublished paper. Undated.

Rossi, P., Freman, H., and Wright, S. *Evaluation: A Systematic Approach.* Beverly Hills,CA: Sage Publication, Inc., 1979.

Rossi, R., Gilmartin, K., and Dayton, C. *Agencies Working Together, A Guide to Coordination and Planning,* Sage Human Services Guide, 28, Beverly Hills, CA: Sage Publications, 1982.

Sandoval, J. *Impact 88: Dallas' Countywide Plan for Reducing Teen Pregnancy,* SIECUS Report 16:5 1-5, 1988.

Scales, P. "Offset Outrage: Let Parents Help Plan." *The American School Board Journal,* p. 32-33, July 1982.

Sonenstein, F. and Pittman, K. "The Availability of Sex Education in Large City School Districts." *Family Planning Perspectives,* 16:19-25, 1984.

Sudman, S. and Bradburn, N. *Asking Questions: A Practical Guide to Questionnaire Design.* San Francisco, CA: Jossey-Bass Inc., 1982.

Task Force on Human Sexuality Education. *Lifespan Human Sexuality Education: Building a Program for the Congregation.* Columbus, OH: The American Lutheran Church, 1986.

The Adolescent Pregnancy Interagency Council. *A Coordinated Strategy on the Issues of Adolescent Pregnancy and Parenting in New York City.* The Mayor's Office of Adolescent Pregnancy and Parenting Services, April, 1986.

Veney, J. and Kaluzny, A. *Evaluation and Decision Making for Health Services Programs.* Englewood Cliffs, NJ: Prentice-Hall, Inc., 1984.

Vincent, M., Clearie, A., and Schlucheter, M. "Reducing Adolescent Pregnancy Through School and Community-Based Education." *Journal of American Medical Association* 257: 3382-3386, 1987.

Wilson, S. *Creating Family Life Education Programs in Public Schools: A Guide for State Education Policymakers*. Alexandria, VA: National Association of State Boards of Education, 1985.

Windsor, Richard A., Baranowski, T., Clark, N., and Cutter, G. *Evaluation of Health Promotion and Education Programs*. Palo Alto, CA: Mayfield Publishing Company, 1984.

Yankelovich Clancy Schulman. *Time/Yankelovich Clancy Schulman Poll: Findings on Sex Education*. New York, 1986.

Zabin, L., Hirsch, M., and Smith, E. Evaluation of a Pregnancy Prevention Program for Urban Teenagers. *Family Planning Perspectives*, 18:119-126, 1986.

Zelnik, M. and Young, J. "Sex Education and Its Association with Teenage Sexual Activity, Pregnancy and Contraceptive Use." *Family Planning Perspectives* 14:117-126, 1982.

For more information on print and video materials developed by
the Stanford Center for Research in Disease Prevention, please write:

Health Promotion Resource Center
Stanford University
1000 Welch Road
Palo Alto, CA 94304-1885
(415) 723-0003

Cover, book design and production: David Collins
Production assistance: Donna Adelman, Meg Babcock